WHY STOMACH ACID IS GOOD FOR YOU

WHY STOMACH ACID IS GOOD FOR YOU

Natural Relief from Heartburn, Indigestion, Reflux, and GERD

Jonathan V. Wright, M.D., and Lane Lenard, Ph.D.

M. Evans and Company, Inc.
New York

M. Evans and Company, Inc.
216 East 49th Street
New York, New York 10017

Library of Congress Cataloging-in-Publication Data

Wright, Jonathan V.
    Why stomach acid is good for you : natural relief from heartburn, indiges-
tions, reflux & GERD / Jonathan Wright and Lane Lenard.
       p.   cm.
    Includes bibliographical references and index.
    ISBN 0-87131-931-4
    1. Achlorhydria—Popular works. 2. Gastric acid—Popular works. 3.
Indigestion—Popular works. I. Lenard, Lane. II. Title.
RC840.A25 W75 2001
616.3'32—dc   2001023343

Typesetting by Evan Johnston

Printed in the United States of America

9   8   7   6   5   4   3   2   1

DISCLAIMER

The ideas and advice in this book are based upon the experience and training of the author and the scientific information currently available. The suggestions in this book are definitely not meant to be a substitute for careful medical evaluation and treatment by a qualified, licensed health professional. The author and publisher do not recommend changing or adding medication or supplements without consulting your personal physician. They specifically disclaim any liability arising directly or indirectly from the use of this book.

for my wife Holly
and with special thanks to June Perbohner,
for her incredible dedication to finding and preserving copies of hundreds of
research papers concerning stomach acid and disease from the 1800s onward
also, thanks to Lane Lenard, Ph.D., coauthor extraordinaire
and Jennifer Morganti, N.D., for her longtime skillful help in the library
and deepest appreciation to the thousands of individuals suffering from low
stomach acid with whom I have worked at Tahoma Clinic—
with the information gathered from your experiences collected and reported in
this book, many, many others will find help for their own health problems

—Jonathan V. Wright, M.D.

for Phyllis and Katy
you make it all worthwhile

—Lane Lenard, Ph.D.

CONTENTS

PREFACE
Whistling Past the Graveyard

Stomach acid has little or no value to our health. We may not even need it for digestion. Therefore, what's the harm in turning off the acid pumps when our gastric juices start erupting into heartburn and acid indigestion? If it gets rid of the pain and discomfort, why not turn them off for the rest of our lives? Stomach acid? Who needs it?

If this sounds silly, try not to laugh too hard, because it's what most doctors in this country believe. The conventional medical establishment in the United States, thanks in large part to hundreds of millions of advertising, research, and "educational" dollars spent by the pharmaceutical industry each year, has learned to fear the evil stomach acid dragon. How else to explain their zeal for pushing dragon-slaying acid suppressors on a public convinced it is drowning in its own internally-produced acid bath?

Acid-suppressing drugs are a more than seven-billion-dollar-a-year industry in the United States. Yet, this unimaginably large franchise is built on a convenient deception: that virtually eliminating acid from the stomach can only be good for us, and that it will have no consequences today, or tomorrow, or twenty or thirty years from now, when we're still popping potent acid-suppressing pills to control our symptoms of "hyperacidity."

In this book, we emphasize some of the important—even essential—roles that stomach acid plays in digestion. We describe how hydrochloric acid, secreted by special cells in the stomach's lining in reponse to a meal, is a key upstream link in a complex chain of events that culminates in the absorption of vital nutrients that make a long, healthy life possible. Break that chain—by severing the acid link—and the downstream cascade of events required for proper digestion and the continuing health of the gastrointestinal (GI) system—as well as the rest of the body—will be severely impeded.

We also ask an important question: What diseases can emerge when stomach acid secretion is too low for too long? We wish the forces that control conventional medicine would ask this question, but for the most part, they seem uninterested. The fact is they don't really want to know the answer. There is simply too much invested in the myth of "acid indigestion."

Yet the consequences for our health of long-term acid reduction due to disease or aging (known as atrophic gastritis) have been well-known for the better part of a century. What about long-term drug-induced acid-suppression? Based on very limited FDA approved trials, conventional medicine's practitioners and promoters feel comfortable pretending that everything's going to be all right for people taking acid-quenching drugs like Prilosec, Prevacid, and their even more powerful successors for ten, twenty, or thirty years or longer—*if* they live that long!

We think that those who choose to believe this myth have their heads buried firmly in the sand. These are powerful drugs that cause profound changes in the body's chemistry and physiology at a key juncture in the digestive process. They should not be taken casually. Yet the current trend, with the widespread promotion of acid-blocking drugs for ordinary heartburn, is promoting just that.

When it comes to acid blockers, the conventional medical establishment—including groups like the American Medical Association (AMA)—National Institutes of Health (NIH), the various specialty medical associations (e.g., American College of Gastroenterology, ACG) and disease advocacy groups (e.g., International Foundation for Functional Gastrointestinal Disorders (IFFGD), not to mention the two most powerful groups of all, the global pharmaceutical industry and its "in-house" enforcement agency, the U.S. Food and Drug Administration (FDA)—are all whistling (in chorus) past the graveyard. At our peril, they ignore decades of research clearly demonstrating that low stomach acid, whether caused by disease or drugs, is linked to a wide range of serious, chronic, so-called incurable diseases, some of which can be fatal.

Just because "serious" problems have not appeared after only a few years of drug use, there's no guarantee we won't start seeing them—and experiencing them—in a few more years. "Natural" atrophic gastritis typically takes decades to progress to more serious conditions such as ulcer or stomach cancer. Why should we expect acid-blocking drugs to be any different?

If you or someone you love suffers from heartburn or other symptoms of gastric upset, we urge you to ignore the constant barrage of advertising that leads most people—including most doctors—to believe that the only way to treat these disorders is by suppressing acid secretion. More than a century's worth of scientific research confirms that this simply isn't so. What has come to be called—incorrectly—"acid indigestion" is almost always associated, not with too much stomach acid, but with too *little*.

In this book, we propose a *natural* program that in many cases can *cure* "acid indigestion." Instead of drugs that merely *suppress symptoms* by disrupting normal GI function, we tell you how to use a variety of safe, natural, inexpensive substances that work *with* the body's physiology—not against it—to *restore* healthy gastric functioning, heal damaged tissues, *prevent* future disease, and perhaps extend your life.

PROLOGUE
The "Gray Man"

At Tahoma Clinic he was known as the "Gray Man." He got the nickname after Sue, the receptionist, and Barbara, the nurse, agreed that they'd never seen anyone with his skin tones. Anyone could see it. Although he was Caucasian, his visible skin was devoid of any pink tones. He scarcely had any brown hue. Instead, he was a peculiar whitish gray. I've not seen anyone with the same pigmentation before or since.

The sixty-one-year-old Gray Man hadn't come in because he was looking gray, although his wife had mentioned it to him "a time or two." Actually, he explained, he didn't have any symptoms or illnesses; he was just plain tired. *Really tired.*

Further questioning turned up little but the fatigue. In the past, he'd had chronic indigestion and intermittent but persistent heartburn. He noted that both symptoms had gone on for over twenty years, and that he'd taken "plenty of those Tums and Rolaids and other antacids" since his forties. However, he reported he hadn't had any indigestion or heartburn problem at all since he'd started taking that "new prescription acid-blocker stuff, Tagamet," which he'd been taking every day since it came out in 1977. By the time he appeared at the clinic, he guessed he'd been taking the drug every day for seven years.

"You know that stomachs are naturally designed to secrete enough acid to turn even large meals into the equivalent of soup?" I asked.

"Yeah, I know that, I guess, but all my doctors told me that my indigestion and heartburn were due to too much acid. It just made good sense to take something that would knock down the excess acid," he replied.

"Did anyone ever actually measure the amount of acid in your stomach?"

"No . . . but the symptoms sure have gone away since I started the Tagamet."

"And a river will dry up if we stop all the rain. Maybe that's an advantage for a little while if the river has been flooding, but what happens if we stop the rain permanently?"

He thought for a moment. "Permanently?"

"Well, seven years, at least."

"Quite a drought. Nothing'll grow, for sure."

"Right. And if we shut off, or neutralize, our stomachs' natural acidity for more than brief intervals, there's bound to be consequences. First, we don't break down foods as well, and many nutrients—especially essential amino acids, certain minerals, and at least two B vitamins—aren't as available as they're supposed to be. So they don't get absorbed into our bloodstreams, and our cells don't get the normal amounts of nutrients they need to keep them going.

"Second, when that 'acidified soup' empties out of our stomachs into the upper part of the small intestine—the duodenum—it triggers the secretion of hormones that in turn stimulate the pancreas and gallbladder to make, or release, their own digestive secretions, including enzymes, bicarbonate, and bile. Without this 'acid trigger,' these hormones are underproduced, and the subsequent stages in digestion don't work as well as they're supposed to, either. This means that another whole group of nutrients becomes less available to our cells."

"So it's like a cascade of events," said the Gray Man, starting to catch on. "If the acidity isn't there, then other parts of digestion aren't triggered properly, either."

"Exactly, and there may be many other 'cascades' in the digestive stream that we still don't know about that might be affected."

"No wonder I'm tired," he said. "I've been literally drying up a lot of my digestion for years. Why didn't anyone tell me about this?"

"Don't know. It's all right there in the basic textbooks for medical students. But that's not all. The same textbooks list a third consequence of low, or no, stomach acid production. Let's think about it this way: What happens if I add bacteria or parasites to an acid solution in a test tube?"

"Not sure, but I'd guess a lot of them'll die."

"Right. They die. Textbooks of gastroenterology—the medical specialty that concentrates on the digestive system—actually refer to stomach acid as the 'acid barrier' to intestinal tract infection. Also, everyone knows that farther down, the intestines are home to a wide variety of microorganisms—sometimes called intestinal microflora (literally tiny plants)—which help with digestion, secrete a few important vitamins, and generally behave themselves.

"But if the acid-alkaline balance—technically called the 'pH'—isn't just right, then many of these 'friendly' microorganisms literally die out and are replaced by not-so-friendly germs. At best, these unfriendly microorganisms aren't as helpful to us as the friendly ones. At worst, some of them may excrete substances that are toxic to our own body cells, which are absorbed and spread all around our bodies."

The Gray Man shifted uncomfortably in his chair. "So by keeping my stomach acid low to prevent heartburn, not only have I been semi-starving myself for the last seven years, but also I may be encouraging toxins from my gut to enter my system?"

"Afraid so."

"Could this be why I've been so tired all the time?"

"Very likely. Let's work on restoring your normal digestion as much as possible. We'll try to make up for all those years of malnutrition, and if necessary we'll do something restore your normal gut flora. Then we'll see what happens with your fatigue."

"I guess the first thing is to stop this Tagamet. But then I'll have indigestion and heartburn all over again, won't I?"

"There are natural ways we can try to stop indigestion and heartburn without blocking stomach acid."

"How?"

"First, we need to find out if your stomach really is making too much acid. Chances are very high—over 90 percent—that the real culprit is likely *underproduction* of stomach acid. Heartburn means that some of that small amount of acid is turning up in the wrong place, causing the burning feeling. Let's wait until we do a test or two."

Like the overwhelming majority of people with indigestion and heartburn, the Gray Man soon found that although he had been suffering from heartburn for years, his stomach had actually been *underpro-*

ducing acid all that time. By replacing the missing stomach acid with capsules containing betaine hydrochloride (a safe, convenient, inexpensive source of stomach acid, or hydrochloric acid—HCl) and the digestive enzyme pepsin with every meal, he was soon able to eliminate his symptoms. His program also included replacement digestive enzymes, intestinal flora normalizers (also called probiotics), and supplements of various amino acids, vitamins, and minerals that he had not been absorbing properly due to his low acid condition.

Slowly but surely, his gray skin color returned to normal, healthy-looking brown and pink skin tones. His fatigue dissipated, too, replaced by increasing energy. His wife also noted an improvement in his mood and attitude. Six months later, he declared himself back to normal.

The only thing entirely atypical about the Gray Man's—John's—case was his skin color. As noted above, I've never seen anything like it before or since. But the rest of his story—indigestion and heartburn caused by *underproduction* of normal stomach acid—is absolutely typical. Since the 1970s, I've worked with literally thousands of individuals with one or another variation of the same story—indigestion and heartburn, frequently accompanied by bloating, belching, gas, constipation, occasionally loose bowels—caused by a failure or partial failure of normal stomach function. (Stomach *overfunction*, or excess acid production, is actually quite rare.) Most of these individuals had been compounding their health problems by taking antacids or acid-blocking drugs either on their own or on the advice of health care practitioners.

In the pages that follow, Dr. Lenard and I explain normal stomach function and what it does for us, and describe some of the many manifestations of "stomach failure." We cover health problems commonly associated with poor stomach function. We describe conventional treatments for the mythical illness known as "acid indigestion," and then the preferred natural alternatives.

As you'll soon find, this is more than just another book about indigestion. For many of us, this is also a for-real guide to antiaging and longevity: *How can we expect our cells and our whole bodies to "live long and well" if they're chronically malnourished?*

For others, we offer a little-known perspective on a variety of diseases, including depression, diabetes, osteoporosis, rheumatoid arthritis, lupus, ulcerative colitis, acne rosacea, multiple sclerosis, childhood asthma, and many others, that often improve once digestive function is normalized.

So why haven't more of us heard about this before? Here's a small clue: The market for antacids and acid-blocking drugs amounts to more than *$7 billion* per year. The actual facts about digestive failure are literally drowned in the sea of advertising and patent medicine (pharmaceutical) industry-sponsored research designed to sustain the profits made from this superficial and profoundly misguided "treatment" of indigestion, heartburn, and accompanying symptoms.

For the *true story,* we invite you to read on!

CHAPTER 1
The Myth of Acid Indigestion

Heartburn, indigestion, dyspepsia, and "acid indigestion" are extremely common afflictions. Thanks mostly to diet and lifestyle, and sometimes because of genetics, pregnancy, anatomy, or simple aging, it seems that sooner or later, almost everybody gets an upset stomach in one form or another. Who hasn't felt the acute burning in the back of the throat and upper chest after eating certain foods? Who hasn't popped a Tums or gulped a "bicarb" to extinguish the acidic flames that seem to roar up from the stomach during a heartburn attack?

A Gallup Poll found that 44 percent of the U.S. population suffers from heartburn at least once a month, and 7 percent experience it weekly.[1] According to the National Institute of Diabetes and Kidney Digestive

Diseases, sixty million people experience heartburn at least once a month and twenty-five million feel the burn every day.

If we are to believe what we see in the media, the American populace is awash in indigestion-causing stomach acid. We can't watch TV (especially the evening newscasts) without seeing dozens of slick commercials for expensive, high-tech drugs like Prilosec, Prevacid, Tagamet, Zantac, Pepcid, Axid, and others, not to mention more traditional low-tech remedies like Tums, Rolaids, Maalox, and Alka-Seltzer. All of these products are designed to eliminate heartburn pain by reducing the amount of acid in the stomach. The old-fashioned antacid remedies simply *neutralize* any acid present in the stomach, taking the acidic "bite" out of it, thus rendering it temporarily harmless. (One popular neutralizing antacid used to advertise that it "soaked up 47 times its weight in *excess* stomach acid.") The more advanced drugs work by squelching the production of acid at its source. The drug most commonly prescribed for heartburn today, Prilosec, virtually eliminates acid in the stomach around the clock, a fact that is proudly promoted in the drug's widespread consumer-oriented advertising. Prevacid, Aciphex, Protonix, and Nexium do about the same thing.

The myth that underlies the conventional treatment of "acid indigestion," and the implied message in all these commercials—although they rarely come right out and say it—is that heartburn happens because we've got *too much acid* in our stomachs. As a result, some of that acid flows back—or *refluxes*—into the esophagus, the muscular tube that carries food from the back of the mouth into the stomach. Since acid does not belong in the esophagus, its presence irritates the delicate tissue that lines the inside of the tube. Heartburn pain is a *symptom* of that irritation. If we've got heartburn or other symptoms of the more serious disorder, *gastroesophageal reflux disease* (GERD), the commercial message is clear: "The less acid we have in our stomachs, the better." To most physicians, it is "common knowledge" that heartburn and other symptoms of acid indigestion are signs of *too much stomach acid*. To relieve the pain, we need merely reduce the level of acid. If we believe this, it makes sense that we should all be using these powerful acid-reducing treatments to relieve our heartburn. According to the manufacturers of these products, long-term acid suppression is an advantage, allowing us to control heartburn "*around the clock,*" perhaps with a single pill.

But as we explain in this book, this kind of extreme heartburn protection may come at a cost to health that is being ignored by the pharmaceutical companies that patent and profit from these drugs, and ignored by the Food and Drug Administration (FDA), which collects truly enormous sums of money to "approve" them. Most importantly, perhaps, the cost to

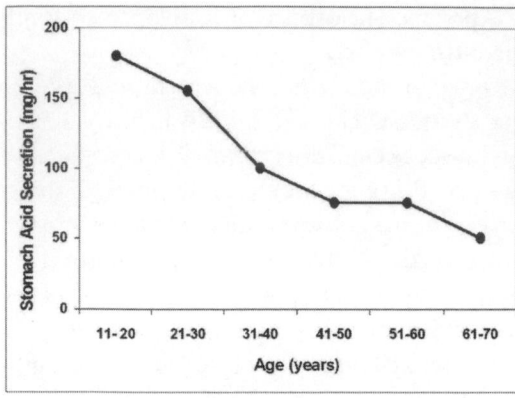

Figure 1-1. Contrary to popular belief, stomach acid secretion tends to decline with advancing age. This graph shows mean stomach acid secretion from the second decade to the eighth decade. Adapted from K. Krentz et al., 1984.

health of these drugs is being ignored by the thousands of physicians who prescribe them. They fail to recognize that the acid-suppression theory, which currently governs the conventional medical therapy of "acid indigestion," is seriously flawed because it is based on the myth that "acid indigestion," heartburn, and its more serious consequence, GERD, are the result of too much stomach acid. The facts say otherwise.

Consider this conveniently overlooked observation: The incidence of indigestion, "simple" heartburn, and GERD *increases* with age, while stomach acid levels generally decline with age (see Figure 1-1). If too much acid were causing these problems, teenagers should have frequent heartburn, while Grandma and Grandpa should have much less. Of course, as everyone knows, exactly the opposite is generally true.

We are led to believe that if we simply have other feelings of *in*digestion, like "that overfull feeling," with excess gas, bloating, or belching, but perhaps only a little heartburn, this is also due to "too much acid." If this is true, then answer this question: Why is *too much* acid so *efficient* at refluxing back into the esophagus but so *inefficient* at actually digesting food?

It is simply a matter of common sense. How many of us can run faster at age forty than at age twenty? How many have better vision at fifty than at thirty? We all experience declining hormone levels as we grow older. We can think of literally dozens of examples of functions that decline naturally with age, so why should the output of acid by the stomach run in the opposite direction? Science has confirmed what common sense tells us. For most of this century, medical researchers have repeatedly and consistently documented an age-related *decline* in stomach acid. So, if we have less and less stomach acid as the years add up, why do we get more and more heartburn and indigestion? And more importantly, why are we treating that heartburn and indigestion by taking drugs that wring the last few drops of acid out of our stomachs?

What's so bad about depleting stomach acid? Lots. Unfortunately, conventional medical wisdom refuses to recognize this, which suits the makers of acid-depleting drugs just fine. The problem is that many of the adverse effects associated with long-term suppression of stomach acid may take years or even decades to develop. At the same time, clinical trials of most drugs, which might expose these problems, generally last only a few months. A year is a long time in the world of clinical trials, and the number of people who take these drugs during these trials is relatively small. Once clinical trials end and a drug is approved by the FDA, monitoring of adverse side effects tends to be relatively haphazard, usually depending on doctors taking the trouble to file reports to the FDA. If a side effect is not immediately and obviously linked to stomach or digestive function, it will probably never get reported. Regrettably, many of the potential accompaniments of long-term acid suppression, including asthma, allergies, skin disorders, rheumatoid arthritis, insomnia, osteoporosis, gastrointestinal (GI) infection, depression, and many, many others, can take years or even decades to develop. They would *seem* to have nothing to do with stomach acid and, therefore, would rarely, if ever, be reported.

GERD: The Serious Side of Heartburn

It wasn't too long ago that heartburn was viewed as largely a nuisance, something we joked about, put up with, blamed on Mother's cooking. Today, heartburn is widely seen by the medical profession as the primary symptom of a potentially dangerous medical condition known as gastroesophageal reflux disease, or GERD. This shift in attitude has been driven in part by new research and partly by the availability (and marketing) of new drugs and surgical procedures.

GERD is not really a disease, per se, but more like a syndrome consisting of one or more of these disorders:

- Damage to the esophageal lining that may or may not produce symptoms.
- Mild to severe inflammation of the delicate lining of the esophagus.
- Symptoms such as heartburn; belching; upset stomach, bloating/gas; sense of fullness, particularly when accompanied by chronic cough; regurgitation of stomach contents, hoarseness, wheezing or asthma, difficulty swallowing, or sore throat.

When heartburn occurs regularly for months or years, it is said to be *chronic*. People with chronic heartburn may have damage to their esophageal lining (especially the lower end of the esophagus) that begins as mild irritation but may end up with scarring, constriction, ulceration, and ultimately, in a very small percentage of people, cancer. This is why intermittent or minor heartburn should never be allowed to become chronic.

Although GERD occurs only in a minority of people who have heartburn, given the potential danger of chronic heartburn, today's acid-trumping treatments would seem to be among modern medicine's more important, if underappreciated, marvels. GERD appears to have met its match in these potent drugs that not only relieve heartburn, but promise to protect us against more serious, even life-threatening conditions.

It's no wonder they have become among the best-selling drugs ever produced. Indigestion/heartburn/GERD is a multibillion-dollar cash cow for the pharmaceutical industry. In the United States alone, we spent more than $7 billion on them in 1999. Prilosec alone accounted for more than half of that, $4 billion, nearly doubling its sales from the previous year.[2]

Indigestion and Heartburn Are Not Caused by Too Much Stomach Acid

As you might have guessed, we think there's something dreadfully wrong with this rosy financial picture. We wonder why so much of humanity is going to such great lengths to rid itself of all that annoying stomach acid, when *very few of us ever consistently has too much acid in our stomachs*, and when (except for a few rare conditions) heartburn is hardly ever associated with *too much* stomach acid.

Chronic heartburn sufferers often have their stomachs and esophaguses examined via x-rays and gastroscopes (fiber optic tubes that allow the doctor to look inside the stomach and even take pictures), but in my thirty years of medical practice, not one person who's had these procedures done elsewhere has ever told me that they have also had careful measurements made of their stomach acid production! When we actually measure stomach acid output under careful, research-verified conditions, the overwhelming majority of heartburn sufferers are found to have *too little* stomach acid production.

Yes, you read that correctly. Heartburn almost never signals *too much* acid, and it may often be associated with *too little!*

This is no secret. This is a well-documented, but little-appreciated, medical fact. It has been confirmed in the scientific literature repeatedly and frequently throughout the last one hundred years.

The pharmaceutical companies, who make all those potent acid-suppressing antiheartburn medications, know that heartburn and GERD are not caused by too much acid. Their researchers are very smart, and they read the scientific literature. They are well aware of the kinds of stomachs their drugs are going into. That's why their ads almost never actually come out and state that heartburn is a proven result of "*too much* acid." Still, the message comes through loud and clear: If stomach acid causes heartburn, then less acid must be better than more.

Logical as this sounds, though, it simply isn't true! As we show in this book, for many people with heartburn and/or GERD, the best treatment may actually be *more acid*, not less. If this sounds like throwing gasoline on smoldering embers, that's right, it does *sound* like it, but in fact, it's not. Paradoxical as it seems, for the better part of a century, knowledgeable physicians have successfully treated tens of thousands of people with indigestion, heartburn, and other diseases related to deficient stomach acid with natural, inexpensive acid supplements (along with various other natural remedies). Once the treatment is completed, indigestion becomes largely a thing of the past, and their patients no longer need to take powerful, expensive, and potentially dangerous (over the long term) acid-suppressing drugs.

Q: When Is a Cause not a Cause?
A: When It "Causes" Heartburn.

Well, one might ask, if heartburn isn't caused by too much acid, then what is it caused by, and why do those drugs seem to work so well? After all, it certainly *appears* that lowering stomach acid levels relieves heartburn and helps heal the esophageal damage associated with GERD.

We do not deny that stomach acid causes the symptoms of heartburn (although not necessarily other forms of indigestion) and that it is responsible for much GERD-related damage. We agree that exposure to acid causes the burning feeling of heartburn, and that chronic exposure to acid can cause more severe conditions such as reflux esophagitis and GERD. Our argument is with the mistaken concept that it takes "too much" stomach acid to do the damage. Even a *small* amount of acid *in the wrong place* (such as the esophagus) can cause symptoms and ultimately tissue damage. (After all, we know that stomach acid must be strong stuff, if it can help reduce even a tough beefsteak into the equivalent of beef soup in an hour or so.)

Nor can we disagree with the fact that lowering the acidity of the stomach often does help relieve the *symptoms* of heartburn and reduce the damage of GERD, albeit temporarily. And yet, we feel quite comfortable in turning around and stating—with absolutely no equivocation—that

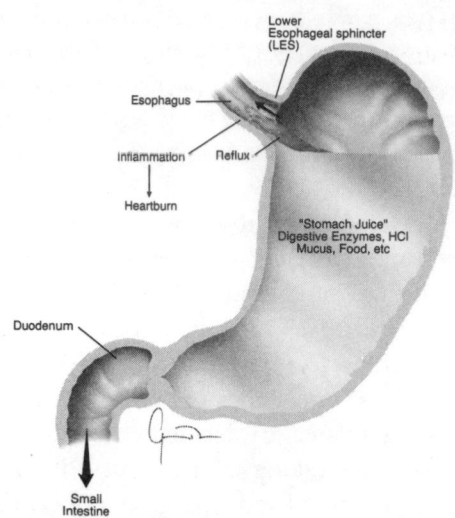

Figure 1-2. Heartburn happens when a small amount of stomach acid refluxes up throught the lower esophageal sphincter (LES) valve, irritating and inflaming the delicate lining of the esophagus.

neither heartburn nor GERD is really *caused* by *too much* stomach acid.

Confused? You're in good company. Most of the medical profession prefers to avoid dealing with this apparent paradox, as well. But is acid taking the heat for the "crime," when its presence in the esophagus is really the result of other events?

As anyone familiar with the relevant scientific literature will quickly agree, heartburn and GERD (but not necessarily the other symptoms of indigestion) are not primarily diseases of stomach acid. Rather they are usually diseases of muscle, specifically the muscular valve (or *sphincter*) that guards the lower end of the esophagus. Known as the *lower esophageal sphincter* (LES), it normally opens wide to permit swallowed food and liquids to pass easily into the stomach, but, except for belching and vomiting, this is the *only* time the LES is intended to open. It's supposed to shut down soon after the food has passed, blocking any acidic stomach juices from making the return trip up the esophagus. If the LES is working properly, it doesn't matter how much acid we have in our stomachs. It's not going to make it up into the esophagus. On the other had, if the LES is asleep at the switch, even a small amount of acid could reflux into the esophagus under the right conditions.

Scientists have found that when we have heartburn or GERD, the LES opens briefly when it's not supposed to. If we've got acid—or anything else—in our stomachs, sometimes even a little bit, and it happens to be in the vicinity of the LES when the valve pops open inappropriately, we get *reflux* (see Figure 1-2). The primary symptom of reflux, of course, is *heartburn*. If reflux happens too frequently and exposes the esophageal lining to too much acid over too long a period, the lining can become irritated or inflamed, a condition known as reflux esophagitis. Once an area has become inflamed or irritated, acid—any amount of acid—will tend to advance the destructive process, ultimately to GERD and the formation of ulcers or worse.

Is an excess of stomach acid to blame in this scenario? Hardly. Acid, after all, is just a liquid, prey to gravity and the muscular contractions of the stomach and esophagus and destined to passively find its own level.

It doesn't matter how much acid there is in the stomach. As long as the LES stays closed, we won't get heartburn or reflux. (Remember, stomachs are built for the very purpose of containing and working with very strong acid, acid that is one-hundred-thousand times stronger than the acidity of our blood.) Instead of pointing the accusing finger at "excess" stomach acid, we should really be eye-balling that old, asleep-at-the-switch gatekeeper, LES.

Conventional Treatments for Heartburn and GERD

Nearly all currently available conventional treatments for heartburn and GERD are designed to reduce the acidity of the gastric juice. Most of these products can be categorized as either *acid neutralizers* or *acid suppressors/acid blockers*.

Acid Neutralizers

These classic products, commonly referred to as *alkalis*, rely on the fundamental chemical fact of life that acids and alkalis (also called bases) *neutralize*, or cancel each other out (see "Acids, Bases, and pH" on page 29). The active ingredients are typically calcium, sodium, aluminum, or magnesium salts that combine with stomach acid (hydrochloric acid, HCl), to form a "neutral" salt. Since antacids do not affect the secretion of stomach acid, their influence on the gastric acid-base balance (known as the pH) is transient, lasting only until all the antacid molecules are used up. In the meantime, the stomach continues to secrete HCl.

Antacid products are easily available without a prescription and are widely regarded as extremely safe. For occasional use, they can be useful for reducing heartburn and, when used this way, probably will not cause any harm. However, overuse, especially when prolonged, can result in serious problems. The most important adverse effect of acid neutralizers is known as the *milk-alkali* syndrome, which consists of excess calcium in the blood, an elevated blood pH (alkalosis), and, most importantly, kidney failure. Milk-alkali syndrome results most easily from the excessive consumption of milk (high calcium) plus an antacid over a long period of time, but it can also occur by taking excessive calcium-based acid neutralizers alone.

In the days before acid-blocking drugs, the combination of large amounts of milk and antacids was a very common conventional treatment for peptic ulcers. Unfortunately, many of the people who followed this dubious medical advice wound up with milk-alkali syndrome. The incidence of the syndrome dropped off sharply with the introduction of the acid blockers. However, it is starting to rise again as people, especially elderly women, take high doses of antacids made from calcium carbonate (e.g., Tums) as a means of supplementing their calcium intake in an attempt to prevent the bone-wasting disease osteoporosis.[3-5] (As we describe in chapter 4, calcium carbonate is one of the worst dietary sources of calcium, because the calcium is so poorly absorbed, especially when stomach acid secretion is low. Since calcium carbonate neutralizes HCl, it actually inhibits the absorption of calcium.)

Other types of antacids contain the metal aluminum. Although the evidence is far from conclusive, it is possible that aluminum may be involved in the development of brain dementias, such as Alzheimer's disease. For safety's sake, it's probably best to avoid the long-term use of these products for this reason alone. Commonly available neutralizing antacids include:

- Aluminum hydroxide + magnesium carbonate (Duracid)
- Aluminum hydroxide + magnesium hydroxide + calcium carbonate (Tempo)
- Aluminum hydroxide + magnesium hydroxide (Maalox, Mylanta, Gelusil, Gaviscon)
- Aluminum hydroxide (Amphojel)
- Aluminum magnesium hydroxide sulfate (Riopan)
- Calcium carbonate + magnesium carbonate (Mi-Acid Gelcaps, Mylanta Gelcaps, Mylagen Gelcaps)
- Calcium carbonate + magnesium hydroxide (Rolaids)
- Calcium carbonate (Tums)
- Magnesium hydroxide (milk of magnesia
- Sodium bicarbonate ("bicarb," baking soda, Alka Seltzer*, Bromo Seltzer)

Acid-Suppressors

Acid blocking drugs come in two basic varieties: *histamine H_2-receptor blockers and proton pump inhibitors.*

Histamine H_2-receptor blockers. These drugs (also called *H_2-blockers*) reduce acid levels by throwing a roadblock right in the middle of the

---

*Alka Seltzer also contains aspirin, which does nothing to relieve heartburn and may irritate the stomach lining.

process that leads to acid secretion. As described in greater detail in chapter 3, most gastric acid secretion is the end result of a process that begins with the hormone gastrin stimulating histamine-producing cells, which in turn signal acid-producing cells to secrete HCl. By blocking the action of histamine, the message never gets to the acid-producing cells to secrete acid. These drugs can be very effective in turning off most of the acid flow for hours at a time.

Originally developed primarily to treat peptic ulcers, they came to be widely used for relieving heartburn/GERD once it became clear that peptic ulcers were actually caused by the bacteria *Helicobacter pylori*, not by excess acid. As their patents ran out, the respective pharmaceutical companies have all brought out low-dose versions of their drugs for nonprescription sales.

As we discuss throughout this book, the long-term, continuous suppression of gastric acid secretion may have important adverse consequences for our health, which are largely ignored by practitioners of conventional medicine. In addition to these effects, these drugs all have well-documented adverse side effects, most of which involve GI disturbances such as constipation, diarrhea, nausea, vomiting, and, yes, heartburn. Tagamet is particularly problematic because it interacts with so many other drugs, producing various adverse effects depending on the other drug. One of the most disturbing of these side effects is an interference with the metabolism of the hormones estradiol (the most potent of the estrogens) and testosterone. In some men, this has resulted in breast enlargement and sexual dysfunction.[6] Currently available H_2-receptor blockers include:

- Cimetidine (Tagamet)
- Ranitidine (Zantac)
- Famotidine (Pepcid)
- Nitazidine (Axid)

Proton Pump Inhibitors. The mechanism inside certain cells in the stomach's lining that actually produces and secretes HCl is known as the *proton pump*. The most potent of the acid-suppressing drugs block the action of this pump mechanism, hence their name, *proton pump inhibitors (PPIs)*. Just one of these pills is capable of reducing stomach acid secretion by 90 to 95 percent for the better part of a day. Taking higher and/or more frequent doses of PPIs, as is often recommended for "intractable" heartburn or for treating peptic ulcers, produces a state of *achlorhydria* (virtually no stomach acid). In addition to the consequences of chronic acid-suppression, there are many serious concerns associated with the use of PPIs.

The most common adverse effects include diarrhea, skin reactions, and headache, which can sometimes be severe.[7-9] Other adverse effects, which occur less frequently, include impotence, breast enlargement,[10] and gout.[11] As we discuss in subsequent chapters, these and other adverse effects directly related to profound suppression of gastric acid secretion by these drugs are a major concern that is being completely ignored by practitioners and supporters of conventional medicine. Currently available proton pump inhibitors include:

- Omeprazole (Prilosec)
- Lansoprazole (Prevacid)
- Rabeprazole (AcipHex)
- Esomeprazole (Nexium)
- Pantoprazole (Protonix)

Motility Enhancers. Drugs known as *motility enhancers* try to tighten up the LES and hustle food (and acid) out of the stomach faster. This would seem to make a little more physiological sense in terms of the actual cause of heartburn, but these drugs have been limited by their unwanted side effects. The most advanced of these drugs, Propulsid, was pulled from the market by the FDA after a few years of widespread clinical use showed that it was causing an unacceptable number of potentially fatal heart failures. As happens all too frequently with new drugs, these problems were not apparent during clinical trials of the drug, but they showed up once the drug was released to the general public and millions of people started using it.

Why Do Anti-Acid Drugs Seem to Work?

Instead of strengthening the LES "dam" and helping it to perform its normal function, conventional medicine treats heartburn/GERD primarily by

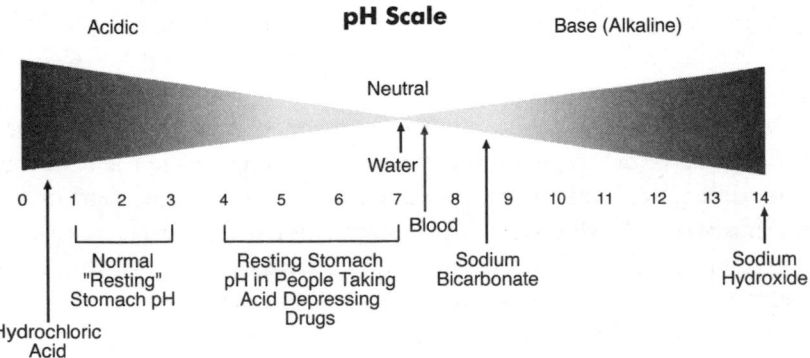

Acids, Bases, and pH

Acids and bases (or *alkalis*) [Pronounced, *AL*-KUH-LIES] are the yin and yang of the chemical world. Scientists measure the relative acidity-alkalinity of a substance by using a *pH* scale. The pH scale ranges from 0 (most acid) to 14 (most alkaline). A pH of 7 is considered neutral.

A common way to measure pH is using strips of litmus or pH paper, which are treated with a chemical that changes color depending on the relative acidity/alkalinity of the substance it contacts. Electronic pH meters that give a numerical readout are typically used when a rapid, precise reading is required.

The HCl produced in the stomach has a pH of 0.8, which makes it an extremely potent acid. HCl is formed in the lining of the stomach by the combination of ions of hydrogen (H+) and chloride (Cl–).

A similarly powerful alkaline substance, like *sodium hydroxide* (also known as lye, or NaOH), has a pH approaching 14. Get this stuff on your hands and you could get just as bad a burn as if you'd handled pure HCl. Because NaOH is so corrosive, it is widely used to unclog bathroom and kitchen drains, selling as Drano and other brand names. Another familiar, but much more benign, alkaline substance is *sodium bicarbonate*, also known as *baking soda*.

In general, our bodies tend to prefer chemicals more toward the *neutral* middle of the pH scale. Water, for example, has a pH of 7, squarely in the middle. Blood tends to be slightly alkaline (pH 7.4). The pH of the "resting," or between-meal, stomach usually ranges from 1 to 3.

When we mix chemical opposites like acids and bases, they tend to *neutralize* each other. Let's say we mix two powerful pH opposites like HCl and NaOH. [Please don't try this at home!] The resulting chemical reaction produces $NaCl + H_2O$, better known as table salt + water, or saline, which has a pH of 7.

One of the earliest means people came up with to relieve heartburn was to swallow an alkaline substance in order to neutralize the offending stomach acid. Of course, we wouldn't want to swallow lye, but sodium bicarbonate works very well, producing not only salt water, but also the gas carbon dioxide (CO_2). The CO_2 can make us feel bloated and cause burping, as it fills the stomach and escapes back up the esophagus.

mopping up as much of the acid "flood" as possible (with neutralizing antacids) or by drying up the river of acid itself (with drugs like Zantac and Prilosec). In so doing, the clinical effects of the malfunctioning LES are are minimized.

To the degree that they reduce the amount of acid available to reflux, these drugs can temporarily relieve the *symptoms* of heartburn and also prevent the damage associated with GERD. Neutralizing antacids reduce gastric (stomach) acidity only modestly, but usually enough to relieve heartburn discomfort for an hour or two. The more potent acid-suppressing drugs reduce the acid secretion by up to 90 percent or more, essentially eliminating acid from the stomach for up to twenty-four hours or longer.[12]

If Symptoms Disappear, What's So Bad About Suppressing Stomach Acid?

Acid-neutralizing agents and acid-suppressing drugs minimize heartburn symptoms, reduce the risks of GERD, can help heal ulcers, and are generally considered by conventional medicine to be safe. Does it really matter that they suppress stomach acid so much? What's the harm? We believe it does matter, for several important reasons:

- The drugs disrupt the natural gastrointestinal environment. Although widely believed to be safe and well tolerated, acid-blocking drugs, by their very nature, induce profound changes in the internal environment of the stomach and intestines. Decades of research have demonstrated that chronically low levels of stomach acid (not necessarily caused by drugs) can be harmful in the long run, leading to maldigestion, malabsorption, and malnutrition, which can predispose to a wide range of serious ailments.

- The relief anti-acid drugs offer is transient. Heartburn stays away only as long as acid levels stay suppressed, and acid levels stay suppressed only as long as we keep taking the drugs. If we stop taking them, we risk heartburn's return, sometimes with a vengeance. It's not uncommon for people to take acid blockers, and even acid neutralizers daily for years and years at a time in order to avoid a relapse.

- The drugs don't cure heartburn, they only temporarily relieve the symptoms. Like many of the "wonder drugs" that have become available in this age of pharmaceutical-dominated medicine, neither acid-blocking drugs nor traditional neutralizing antacid products do anything to cure heartburn or GERD. They only temporarily suppress the major symptom—heartburn. Symptom suppression is the standard treatment strategy for most diseases in conventional Western medicine today. With the possible exception of antibiotics, very few drugs being marketed today can actually cure anything.

- These drugs may be effective at removing the irritating agent, but as far as the cause is concerned, they completely miss the point. We can think of acid-blocking treatment like drying up the river after a flood but never repairing the faulty dam that's actually causing the flooding. Note how gingerly the American College of Gastroenterology (ACG) treats the issue of "cure" (see below). Although they use the "c-word" rather loosely, it's clear that, from their conventional perspective, the only "real" cure is not drugs but surgery.

- We can become dependent, or at least *reliant,* on anti-acid drugs. They work only as long as we keep taking them. Stopping treatment commonly triggers an acid "rebound," which can be quenched only by—you guessed it—taking more acid suppressing drugs. Although the rebound is typically short-lived, lasting a couple of days at most,

Can Anything Actually Cure My Troubling Heartburn?
What the American College of Gastroenterology says:

"In patients with mild heartburn, simple lifestyle changes may improve symptoms. However, patients with more severe symptoms or esophageal damage usually need either long-term medications or surgery to *cure* their heartburn. Similar to the treatment of high blood pressure, *medications for GERD control the disease, but are effective only when taken regularly.* For those who cannot achieve adequate symptom relief and healing through medical therapy, *anti-reflux surgery offers the only potential for cure by strengthening the lower esophageal sphincter.*" (Italics added.)

—Patient Information

---

*Even the "curative" powers of antibiotics are debated by natural medicine practitioners. Continuing the classic "Bechamp vs. Pasteur" argument of the nineteenth century, many agree with Bechamp that infection is only a symptom of an underlying weakness or disorder of the immune system, which antibiotics do nothing to cure.

how many people are willing to "tough it out" and endure the heartburn when they can quickly squelch it by getting back on their acid blocker? While this isn't exactly a true addiction, once this cycle gets going, we're almost as good as "hooked" on acid suppression.

This strategy leaves much to be desired for people with heartburn, but it works great for the pharmaceutical companies. If the drugs actually cured heartburn/GERD, the companies wouldn't make nearly as much money as they do by selling drugs that provide only temporary symptomatic relief.

Repairing the Cause of Indigestion and Heartburn, the Natural Way

A much more sensible—but less profitable—tactic is to treat the *root cause* of the problem, repair it, and send us on our way, heartburn- and indigestion-free, and unbeholden to the pharmaceutical gods Prilosec, Zantac, their cousins, and their descendants. Curing a disease means eliminating the cause of the problem. When a disease is cured, it does not return once the treatment is halted. Curing a disease means removing the reason we developed heartburn in the first place, not just suppressing its symptoms.

With treatment that addresses the *cause* of the symptoms, indigestion can almost always be eliminated, and (as a consequence of addressing the cause), overall health improves. Given the right environment and enough time to heal itself, an irritated or injured LES often returns to its normal, healthy state, eliminating heartburn. Even the more severe condition of GERD can often (but not always) be brought under control by this approach to treatment.

All of this can be accomplished by proper diagnosis, elimination of offending agents, food allergies and sensitivities, toxins (including caffeine, nicotine, and alcohol), and then by taking a variety of *natural* substances, including (in almost all cases) supplements of stomach acid (HCl) itself. Applied judiciously at the appropriate times and accompanied by certain dietary and lifestyle modifications, these treatments can help return digestion to normal, restore the GI environment to near normal conditions, eliminating indigestion, heartburn, and even GERD for good.

If this sounds suspiciously like the "c-word," for many people it is. Once their indigestion and/or heartburn/GERD is gone, it's gone. They may no longer need to take some of their natural treatments again, let alone their Prilosec or their Tums. However, people who are found by actual testing to have a stomach acid deficiency (remember, they're the overwhelming majority of those with indigestion) can benefit with better overall health by continuing to take acid supplements with their meals. This particular benign, *natural* solution involves *replacing something the body is missing*. It avoids using synthetic chemicals the body is ill-equipped to handle.

Beyond Heartburn: Treating Other Diseases Related to Low Stomach Acid

As a physician practicing for more than thirty years, I've seen the harm that low stomach acid can do over a long period of time. I have worked with thousands of patients who arrived at the Tahoma Clinic with diseases as disparate as rheumatoid arthritis, childhood asthma, type 1 diabetes, osteoporosis, chronic fatigue, depression, and many others only to find that they all had one thing in common: their stomachs were putting out a less-than-optimal amount of acid. In many cases, by restoring normal gastric function using safe, inexpensive acid supplements; pepsin and other digestive enzymes; and amino acids, vitamins, minerals, and botanicals, we have been able to help them improve or even eliminate their disease conditions. And we do this with almost no risk of dangerous side effects.

Admittedly, the idea that heartburn and other diseases may be related to too little stomach acid and can be treated by swallowing more acid flies in the face of medicine as it is taught and practiced today. This wasn't always the case. Hardly anyone pays any attention to the medical facts—many of them accumulated during the 1920s, 1930s, and 1940s—showing that low stomach acid occurs disproportionately in people with numerous serious diseases. This is old science, but it is still good science, and most of these findings are just as valid today as they were then. However, no matter what their age, such ideas do not fit comfortably into conventional medical wisdom, much of it propagated by the pharmaceutical companies in support of their valuable acid-suppressing drugs. The multibillion-dollar anti-acid franchise depends on the conventional medical wisdom staying right where it is.

Yet, the truth is that correcting digestive malfunction can often yield dramatic improvements in many of these diseases. Remarkably, in children with asthma, it can be part of the cure. In hundreds of cases, I have found that more than 50 percent of children who come to me with asthma can have their wheezing *cured* simply by normalizing their stomach acid and properly administering vitamin B_{12}, with no bronchodilators and no corticosteroids. Think about that: *curing the wheezing of childhood asthma!* There is no conventional pharmaceutical treatment for asthmatic wheezing on the market that can even come close to permanently eliminating the most life-threatening symptom of this disease.

The fact is that the corticosteroids and bronchodilators people with asthma commonly take—often daily for their entire lives—do not and cannot cure asthma. Instead of removing the cause of the disease, they merely suppress the symptoms. And to make matters worse, they can have serious side effects.

This is not a pretty picture, but it is an accurate depiction of the way most doctors treat childhood asthma today. Unfortunately, their treatment strategies are based on a fundamental misunderstanding of the nature of most childhood asthma.* The cause of asthma in these children lies not in their airways, but in their stomachs. Certainly, treating the symptoms (wheezing, bronchial inflammation) provides quick temporary relief, but it does nothing to eliminate the cause. Instead, it may leave the child "reliant" on dangerous and costly drugs until the asthma "disappears" (as it often does) at puberty, or even possibly for the rest of his or her life. By treating the causes, the symptoms often resolve without further treatment, and they do not return as long as stomach acid is kept at an optimum level and vitamin B_{12} is supplied. This is why we have been able to *cure* the wheezing of half of all the children who come to our clinic with asthma. (We realize that children with asthma *have not* been taking the antacids or acid blockers we've been discussing. We mention this condition as an example of one of the many diseases associated with inherently low levels of stomach acid that can be improved or cured by appropriate attention to stomach function.)

It's Your Choice

If you have indigestion or heartburn, or a disease frequently associated with low stomach acid output and poor digestion, which would be preferable, *treat the cause* or take a drug to suppress the indigestion and heartburn, and then more drugs for each other symptom? The answer appears obvious, yet it's going to be a long time before conventional medicine gives up its antacid/acid-blocker cash cow.

Fortunately, you don't have to wait until the FDA, the American Medical Association, and the many other alphabet-soup agencies that control the "conventional wisdom" in medicine today (almost always following the pharmaceutical industry line) see the "error of their ways." (Hint:

---

* This fundamental understanding of the root cause of most childhood asthma is over 300 years old, and (despite my gray hair) didn't originate with me. The very first English-language book devoted to asthma (Floyer, *A Treatise of the Asthma,* 1698) stated that "asthma is a winde arising in the stomache." See chapter 6 for more about origins of asthma in the stomach.

It's never going to happen, because there's so little profit in the natural—unpatentable—acid, vitamin, mineral, amino acid, herbal and other supplements that can be used to eliminate heartburn, and indigestion and to treat related diseases.) You could go down to your local health food store right now and purchase everything you need for a fraction of the cost of filling a prescription for Prilosec, Prevacid, or other acid suppressor.

Before you do that, though, we suggest you read this book first, because you'll learn that:

- The pharmaceutical industry spends billions trying to convince us that "acid indigestion" comes from too much stomach acid, even though a casual reading of the scientific literature on the subject reveals that the opposite is true.

- As we age, stomach acid levels do not increase, as we would expect from the increase in heartburn associated with age. In fact, for most people, acid secretion decreases with age.

- Overuse of neutralizing or buffering antacids, and ordinary use of powerful acid-suppressing drugs, can inhibit the absorption of essential nutrients and impair the digestion of protein, minerals, and a few vitamins.

- The resulting malnutrition can, over many years, lead to depression, osteoporosis, arthritis, and other chronic degenerative diseases that reduce the quality of our lives and may ultimately shorten our life spans.

- The best way to treat "acid indigestion" is not with less stomach acid, but (almost always) with more.

- Replacement acid in the form of safe, inexpensive substitutes for endogenous (internally produced) stomach acid, such as betaine hydrochloride and glutamic acid hydrochloride, enhances digestion, and causes heartburn, indigestion, bloating and gas eventually to vanish.

- The improved digestion and absorption of essential nutrients that result from appropriate acid replacement, combined with natural supplemental digestive enzymes and elimination of toxins and allergens, improves health and reduces the symptoms of a long list of diseases associated with low stomach acid production.

- In many of us, correcting the naturally occurring, gradual "digestive failure of aging" will help restore energy and improve health, thus extending life.

A Note of Caution

Heartburn is usually a benign condition, but if you suffer from it regularly for months or even years at a time, it can be a sign of diseases such as reflux, esophagitis, esophageal ulcer or *Barrett's esophagus*, a serious condition that can lead to a fatal form of cancer. Thus, we always suggest that the first step you take in treating your heartburn is to consult a physician who can rule out the serious diseases and who will then guide and support you in treating your heartburn/GERD the natural way. In the final chapter in this book, we tell you how to find a knowledgeable physician who, when you utter the words "heartburn" or "indigestion" won't automatically reach for the Prilosec.

CHAPTER 2
Why Stomach Acid Is Your Friend

Amidst all the media noise about "acid indigestion" and *too much* stomach acid, it is easy to forget a painfully obvious fact: *Acid is in the stomach because it is supposed to be there*. Acid is not some nuisance substance the stomach uses to punish us for enjoying a pepperoni pizza. Acid plays a variety of vital roles in the digestive process. Without it, our digestive health—and our health in general—is doomed to suffer. This chapter discusses a few of the major roles stomach acid plays.

Acid Promotes the Digestion and Absorption of Many Vital Nutrients

Nutrients such as the peptide and amino acid components of proteins, minerals (including iron, copper, zinc, and calcium), as well as vitamin B_{12}

and folic acid, all depend on adequate stomach acid for their digestion and absorption. Stomach acid accomplishes this by optimizing the gastric pH (the acid/base balance) and by triggering the action of the stomach's own digestive enzyme, pepsin. If, because of inadequate stomach acid, our breakfasts, lunches, and dinners aren't being digested, then we can't absorb the amount of nutrients from that food that Nature intended. How can we expect to stay healthy if we have chronically poor nutrient absorption due to incomplete digestion?

Breaking down whole food into its nutrient components that can be easily absorbed into the bloodstream is the raison d'être of digestion. In many important ways, our stomachs initiate this process. For many essential nutrients, this breakdown occurs at an optimum rate only within a narrow range of relative acidity. If there is too little acid, the normal chemical reactions required to break down and make nutrients ready for absorption may not occur at maximum efficiency. If this condition persists for an extended period of time, a state of selective malnutrition may result that can adversely affect various vital bodily functions, many of them well beyond the digestive system. Over time, this can and does lead to diseases such as anemia, osteoporosis, cardiovascular diseases, depression, and many others. (Our nurses and technicians are always surprised when a woman who is known to have the bone wasting disease osteoporosis—due in part to poor calcium absorption—turns out to have *normal*, rather than low stomach acid.) At the other extreme, too much acid can literally eat away the tissues of the digestive tract, contributing to ulcers. As we have said, though, true long-term hyperacidity is very rare.

Acid Helps Digest Protein by Stimulating Pepsin Production

Pepsin is an enzyme that is required for the optimum initial digestion of protein. During the ingestion of food, the secretion of stomach acid triggers the production of pepsin. If acid levels are depressed, then so are pepsin levels. As a result, proteins don't get broken down into their component amino acids and peptides (two or more linked amino acids). The resulting deficiency of many *essential* amino acids,* including *phenylala-*

---

*Some amino acids (and other nutrients) are termed essential because the body cannot manufacture them itself. They must be obtained from external sources such as food and/or supplements.

nine, and *tryptophan*, as well as the "nonessential" amino acid *tyrosine*, may lead to chronic *depression, anxiety, insomnia,* and other disturbing or dangerous long-term disorders.

At the same time, the proteins that escape digestion by pepsin may find their way into the bloodstream, an event that would not normally happen in a healthy GI tract. The body generally reacts with hostility to the presence of "foreign" proteins in the blood or other tissues. The resulting *immune* response is similar to what happens when the body mobilizes its powerful defenses (e.g., T cells, B cells, and antibodies) to eliminate a viral or bacterial infection. In this way, inadequate digestion by our stomachs (as well as inadequate pancreatic function) can contribute to gradually increasing *food allergies*. For reasons not completely understood, although genetics are a factor, people with autoimmune diseases such as *lupus, rheumatoid arthritis, type 1 diabetes, Graves' disease*, and many others very frequently have low levels of stomach acid, poor digestion, and many food allergies that serve to aggravate their conditions. (The possible role of low stomach acid in autoimmune and related diseases is discussed in greater detail in chapter 6.)

Stomach Acid Prevents Bacterial and Fungal Overgrowth

Here's an extreme, but very revealing, incident: Decades ago, public health officials in India investigated why some people in a village in the midst of a cholera epidemic didn't contract the disease, while others did. They found that many more of those who stayed healthy had normal levels of stomach acid, while those who developed the disease usually did not. Apparently, the strong stomach acid killed the cholera bacteria before it could "colonize" (and damage) the entire gastrointestinal tract.

Most bacteria cannot survive very long in a highly acidic environment. While bacteria are found in abundance in the less acidic regions of the GI tract—the mouth, esophagus, small intestine, and especially the large intestine (colon)—the stomach remains largely sterile due to its natural acidity.

As the acid barrier begins to break down (as can happen after taking acid-blocking drugs or with certain common disease states), the stomach becomes vulnerable to bacterial invasion on two fronts. First, otherwise "friendly" bacteria that normally live comfortably in the small intestine (where they help with digestion) find a more alkaline gastric environment less threatening. They may migrate up to the stomach, where they multiply and colonize the once-forbidden territory.

At the same time, common bacteria constantly—and unavoidably—enter the body through the nose and mouth. Ordinarily, they would quickly meet their maker in a pool of stomach acid, but when stomach acid is deficient, many of these microorganisms may live to multiply—and infect—another day. Most bacteria that enter by these routes are relatively benign. They may interfere with the digestion of some nutrients, and they may cause symptoms like diarrhea, constipation, and stomach pain in some cases, but the disruption is rarely serious. But some microorganisms, including *Salmonella*, certain extremely virulent strains of *E. coli*, and the *Vibrio cholerae* noted above, can cause serious illness, even death, when low stomach acid allows them to gain a beachhead on the gastric shores.

The significance for our health of a strong *acid barrier* in the stomach is discussed in greater detail in chapter 4.

What Happens When Stomach Acid Levels Get Too Low?

Until relatively recently, physicians were concerned, not so much with the effects of *high* levels of stomach acid, but more with the long-term effects of excessively *low* levels. A decline in acid secretion with advancing age has been well documented.[1] From the late nineteenth century to the mid-twentieth century, researchers regularly reported that the number of people with *anacidity* (total or near total absence of stomach acid), also known as *achlorhydria*, and *low acidity,* also called *hypochlorhydria*, increased with age from a low of about 4 percent at age twenty to as much as 75 percent after age sixty. A 1941 reviewer of stomach acid research observed:

> "Anacidity or achlorhydria is more likely to be evidence of disease of the stomach than any other variation of gastric secretion . . . *There is no disease known capable of inducing true gastric hyperacidity** . . . Pathological deviations in acid and pepsin concentrations were *invariably in the direction of decrease.*"[2] (Italics added for emphasis.)

As recently as 1996, a British physician, reviewing age-related GI disorders, noted that stomach acid output commonly declines as people age, due to a loss of the cells that produce the acid. This condition is termed *atrophic*

---

*Rare diseases such as Zollinger-Ellison syndrome, which are associated with excess stomach acid, were unknown in 1941.

gastritis, or *gastric atrophy*. Moreover, a large portion of "normal," healthy people above age sixty—without heartburn—have atrophic gastritis.[3]

Atrophic gastritis is the major cause of "age-related" declining stomach acid levels. Many studies have demonstrated that people with atrophic gastritis are exceptionally vulnerable to a wide range of serious disorders that go far beyond the stomach and esophagus. These include:

- Poor absorption of important vitamins, minerals, and amino acids
- Poor digestion of proteins
- Allergies
- Bronchial asthma in childhood (an obvious exception to "age-relat ed" atrophic gastritis)
- Depression
- Bacterial overgrowth in the stomach and small intestine, leading to symptoms such as heartburn, "gas," constipation, diarrhea, and an increased susceptibility to potentially fatal infections such as cholera and *Salmonella*.
- Pernicious anemia
- Stomach cancer
- Skin diseases, including forms of acne, dermatitis (itching, redness, swelling), eczema, and urticaria (hives)
- Gall bladder disease (gallstones)
- Rheumatoid arthritis
- Lupus erythematosus
- Grave's disease
- Ulcerative colitis
- Chronic hepatitis
- Osteoporosis
- Type 1 (insulin-dependent) diabetes
- Accelerated aging

Functional Gastric Atrophy

If stomach acid is so important, and if chronically low levels of stomach acid can make us chronically sick, does it make any sense to be taking drugs whose sole purpose is to to deplete stomach acid even further?

Scientific studies have so far been unable to show conclusively that taking acid-suppressing drugs contributes to the development of atrophic gastritis. However, there have been reports that taking Prilosec can sometimes lead to achlorhydria that lasted more than two years after discontinuing the drug.[4]

Even without destroying acid-producing cells in the stomach, acid suppressing drugs can create a chronic state that amounts to *functional gastric atrophy*. In other words, both the disease and the drug accomplish the same feat: They drastically reduce stomach acidity to far below normal.

We know what can happen when stomach acid levels are depressed for decades due to ordinary, garden-variety atrophic gastritis. But what happens after decades of depressed stomach acid due to functional gastric atrophy induced by decades of using today's powerful acid suppressors? Nobody knows for sure. Prilosec has been widely used for only a few years. Prevacid, Aciphex, Protonix, and Nexium are even newer. Will we be seeing a rise in the occurrence of stomach cancer, arthritis, osteoporosis, or other serious diseases as these drugs become even more popular and people start entering their second and third decade of continuous drug-induced gastric hypoacidity? We think it's very likely, but to be "scientifically precise," we must say that nobody knows for sure. But why take this risk at all?

CHAPTER 3
How the Upper GI Tract Works . . . Basically

Most of us have only a vague idea of how the digestive system works. We know, for example, that after we put food into our mouths, chew it, and swallow it, it passes into the stomach, and what's left after digestion is complete eventually passes out of the body in the form of a bowel movement. We might remember from high school science classes that the *gastrointestinal (GI) tract*, where digestion occurs, is essentially a hollow tube that begins at the mouth and ends at the anus. Although it is named after its two most prominent features, the *stomach (gastro-)* and the *intestines*, the GI tract actually consists of many more vital structures (see Figure 3-1).

Most of us also have a general idea that what we eat not only comes out the other end, but also finds its way into the rest of our bodies, nourishing bones, muscles, nerves, blood, and every other organ, tissue, and cell. The familiar expression, "You are what you eat," is at least partly true. The food

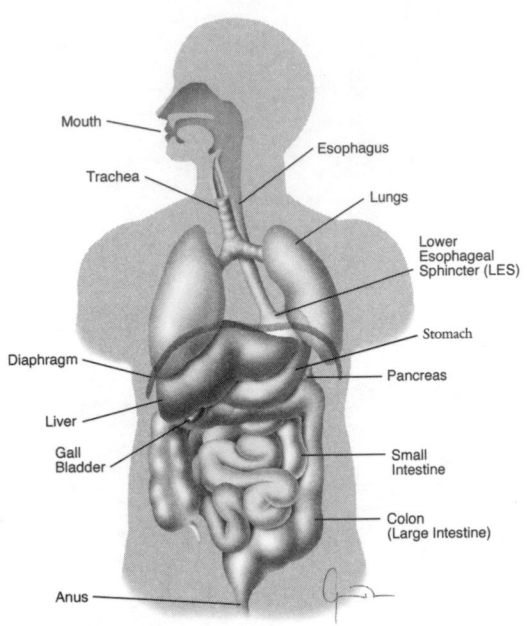

Mouth
Esophagus
Trachea
Lungs
Lower Esophageal Sphincter (LES)
Stomach
Diaphragm
Pancreas
Liver
Gall Bladder
Small Intestine
Colon (Large Intestine)
Anus

Figure 3-1. Major organs of the gastrointestinal system, as well as the lungs, trachea (windpipe), and diaphragm.

we eat gets converted in the GI tract into something that quickly becomes an intimate part of our physical being. Every cell in the body is comprised of materials that began their existence somewhere in the outside world.

Digestion is the process by which food gets broken down in the GI tract by both mechanical and chemical processes, so that nutrients can be *extracted from the food*, *absorbed* into the blood stream, and *distributed* throughout the body for the myriad purposes involved in keeping us alive and kicking.

Although we often take it for granted, digestion involves a highly complex and well-coordinated interaction of many different acids, enzymes, alkaline substances, hormones, and other items too numerous to mention. When these are produced and released in just the right amounts at just the right times, digestion proceeds unnoticed, in the background, perfectly. But if something upsets the balance, say a deficiency in stomach acid, it can have profound health effects that may manifest as an upset stomach or heartburn, but may extend far beyond the stomach itself.

In this chapter, we focus on a small but extremely important part of the digestive story that takes place in the region sometimes called the *upper GI tract*, which includes the mouth, esophagus, and stomach. The upper GI tract functions as a kind of staging area for the digestive system. It is here that food is broken into small, manageable pieces, softened, lubricated, and liquefied. At the same time, proteins, amino acids, minerals, and other nutrients are extracted from food and processed to make them optimally available for the subsequent steps in digestion and absorption that take place later on. Any disruption here will be felt and magnified far downstream. Like most other processes in the body, digestion can be extremely complex, but don't get scared, we'll try to keep it simple.

The Mouth

Digestion begins in the mouth, where the act of chewing breaks down the food into smaller, more manageable pieces and mixes it with *saliva*. Saliva, which is released as soon as food enters the mouth (or even at its sight, smell, or thought, for Pavlov fans), moistens the food and begins the process of

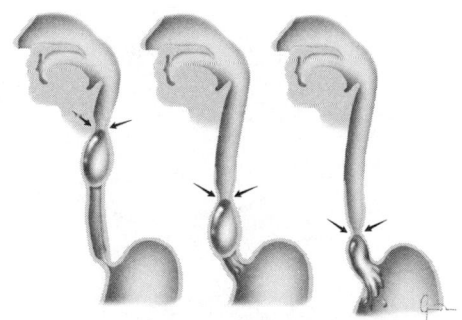

Figure 3-2. The action of peristalsis propels a "bolus" of food from the mouth to the stomach. The LES remains closed until the food approaches the esopheageal-stomach junction, at which point it opens briefly to allow the food to pass through.

breaking down starches. It also helps lubricate the food so it can pass more easily through the next leg of the journey, the *esophagus*.

The Esophagus

The esophagus is a muscular tube that begins in the back of the throat and merges at its lower end with the upper part of the stomach. The esophagus consists basically of a smooth inner tube lined with delicate *epithelial cells*. The inner tube is surrounded by layers of muscle tissue. When we swallow, the esophageal muscle reacts by initiating a rhythmic series of contractions—called *peristalsis*—that start at the top and work their way down toward the stomach (see Figure 3-2). The effect is to propel the food into the stomach. For those who like statistics, it takes about six to eight seconds for a swallow of food to traverse the entire length of the esophagus and enter the stomach. The food proceeds at an average velocity of about one inch per second.

The *LES* is the valve that guards the junction between the esophagus and stomach. As mentioned in chapter 1, in order for food to pass from esophagus to stomach, the LES must relax. It does this quite readily when food reaches the lower end of the esophagus, and it then quickly tightens up, acting as a barrier against the contents of the stomach, which would otherwise *reflux* (literally, "flow back") up into the esophagus. This barrier function is critical, because unlike the stomach, the delicate tissue that lines the inside of the esophagus cannot stand up to the harsh digestive juices normally and naturally present in the stomach.

When the LES is in its normal resting mode, with no swallowing and little or no food in the stomach, its average pressure is about 20 mm Hg

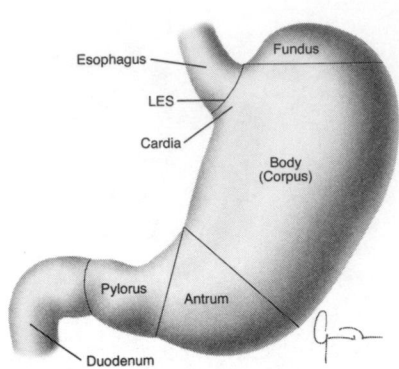

Figure 3-3. Schematic representation of the stomach showing the major regions and connecting organs.

(millimeters of mercury). (This means a counterpressure of 20 mm Hg would have to be applied to pry it open.) About 1.5 to 2.5 seconds after we swallow, LES pressure drops (relaxes) and remains low for six to eight seconds. Stomach contractions that increase pressure in the stomach cause the LES to tighten up to protect the esophagus against reflux.[1]

The problem in heartburn/reflux/GERD is hardly ever low *resting* LES pressure. Researchers have found that reflux usually occurs when little low-pressure blips called *transient LES relaxations* (*TLESRs*) cause LES pressure to fall briefly. TLESRs have nothing to do with swallowing. For reasons medical science does not yet completely understand, they occur all by themselves at intervals that vary from person to person and from hour to hour within the same person. And because most reflux events occur during TLESRs, people who have them frequently also have a higher risk of developing reflux esophagitis or worse.[2]

The Stomach

The stomach is a large, muscular, bladderlike structure, perfectly suited to churning a quantity of chewed and swallowed food, mixing it with potent acids, enzymes, and other digestive juices, and blending these into a liquefied mush called *chyme*.

The stomach is considered to have several major regions, including the *cardia*, *fundus*, *body (corpus)*, *antrum*, and *pylorus*. It connects to the esophagus at its upper end (cardia) and the duodenum at its lower end (pylorus). The duodenum connects the stomach to the small intestine (see Figure 3-3).

The stomach serves four basic functions:

- **Storage reservoir.** It stores swallowed food for a short time. This reservoir function lets us eat a substantial meal in a relatively short time and process it later.

- **Food processing.** It liquefies and grinds the food, mixing it with various digestive juices.

- **Nutrient extraction and digestion.** It begins the extraction and digestion of proteins as well as numerous vitamins and minerals.

- **Transfer.** When the appropriate consistency of stomach contents is reached, the stomach begins feeding chyme through the duodenum into the small intestine, where the major work of digestion and nutrient absorption begins.

The lining of the stomach consists of six basic types of cells, each of which secretes one or more important substances:

- **Parietal cells** secrete HCl, a highly potent acid that participates in many reactions and lowers the intragastric pH (acidity inside the stomach) to the range that is optimal for digestion and absorption of nutrients. As we noted in chapter 1, the cellular mechanism that is principally responsible for the production of stomach acid is known as the proton pump. Drugs known as proton pump inhibitors, turn off this pump, reducing acid secretion by more than 90 percent. Parietal cells also secrete intrinsic factor, which is required for the absorption of vitamin B_{12}.

- **Chief cells** secrete pepsinogens, which are converted with the help of HCL into the protein-busting enzyme pepsin.

- **G cells** secrete gastrin, an extremely important regulatory hormone that regulates the release of HCl from parietal cells and pepsinogens from chief cells. Gastrin also stimulates stomach muscles to contract and promotes the growth of the gastric mucosa (the lining of the stomach).

- **Enterochromaffin-like (ECL) cells** secrete histamine in response to stimulation by gastrin.

- **Mucous cells** secrete mucus, which helps lubricate and liquefy the food. Mucus also helps protect the stomach lining from the caustic intragastric environment.

- **D cells** secrete somatostatin, a hormone that puts the brakes on food processing in the stomach by slowing the rate of gastrin secretion as the intragastric pH falls.

Gastric Acid Secretion

Present scientific knowledge tells us that stomach acid secretion is under the control of three separate substances: *acetylcholine*, *gastrin*, and *histamine*.

- Acetylcholine (ACh) is a neurotransmitter, a hormonelike substance that carries information within the nervous system and between the nerve and muscle cells. Neural control of acid secretion via ACh makes it possible for the stomach to start secreting acid at the sight, smell, or even thought of food, as impulses originating in the brain trigger the release of ACh onto parietal cells.

- Gastrin promotes HCl secretion by two routes: it directly stimulates parietal cells, which respond by pumping out acid molecules. More important is gastrin's ability to stimulate ECL cells to secrete histamine.

- Histamine, in turn, stimulates parietal cells to release HCl. The location on the parietal cell where histamine binds is called the H_2 receptor. Histamine action at the H_2 receptor is the primary stimulus for gastric acid release. Drugs known as H_2-receptor blockers, including Zantac, Tagamet, Pepcid, and Axid, prevent gastrin from stimulating H_2 receptors, which significantly reduces acid release into the stomach.

The Digestive Cascade: What Happens When Food Enters the Stomach?

When a swallow of food passes through the LES and enters the stomach, it triggers a highly coordinated series of events designed to optimize digestion (see Figure 3-4):

- The stomach lining stretches a bit.

- The stretching is sensed by nerve fibers that signal G cells to begin secreting gastrin.

- Gastrin stimulates parietal cells to increase acid secretion and release. It also stimulates ECL cells to secrete histamine, which then stimulates parietal cells to increase acid secretion and release.

- Parietal cells also release a substance known as intrinsic factor, which is required for the absorption of vitamin B_{12}.

- Gastrin also triggers the release of pepsinogens from chief cells in the gastric mucosa.

- Pepsinogens, in the presence of sufficient HCl, are converted into pepsin, the primary stomach enzyme responsible for breaking down proteins into amino acids. (The conversion of pepsinogen to pepsin occurs optimally when the pH of the stomach is 4 or less. If the pH should rise to 5 or higher [less acidic], pepsinogens are inactivated, and no pepsin is formed.)

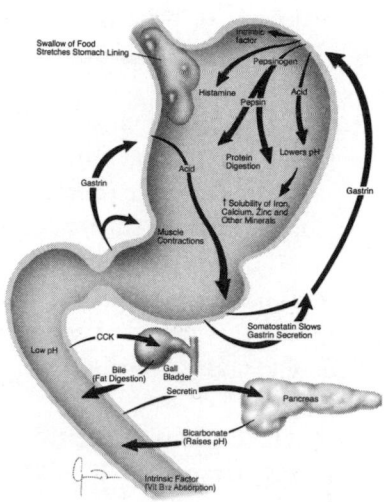

Figure 3-4. The digestive cascade.

- While all this is going on, gastrin also signals the stomach muscles to begin churning and grinding away, helping to mix the contents and to move them along. Once the stomach's contents (chyme) have been "fully acidified," the processing of proteins and many other vitamins and minerals can move ahead at an optimal rate.

- By the time the chyme reaches the lower reaches of the stomach, the pH begins to rise so that the digestion and absorption can take place in the small intestine. The acidity of the stomach is reduced in the lower regions of the stomach—the antrum and pylorus. This occurs by two main mechanisms. First, available acid stimulates D cells in the antrum to begin secreting the hormone somatostatin. Somatostatin feeds back to G cells to slow the production of gastrin. Less gastrin means less histamine and less acid secretion from parietal cells. Second, acidified chyme contacting the lining of the duodenum stimulates the release of the hormone secretin.

- Secretin, in turn, signals the pancreas (a large gland best known for secreting the hormone insulin) to release a variety of digestive enzymes as well as ions of bicarbonate. Bicarbonate produced by the pancreas is actually the same as the "bicarb" that (i.e., sodium bicarbonate, or baking soda) that people have long used to relieve heartburn by neutralizing stomach acid (raising the pH).

- The hormone cholecystokinin (CCK) is released in the small intestine at the same time as secretin. It travels to the gallbladder, where it stimulates the release of bile—essential for the proper digestion of fats—into the small intestine.

This has been a highly simplified description of a vastly more complex process. Nevertheless, it serves to make five extremely important points about acid and GI function:

1. These essential digestive functions can occur only within a very narrow range of pH, and that range shifts depending on the stage of digestion.

2. "Blocking" or "neutralizing" stomach acid interrupts the normal digestive cascade at a crucial juncture. It removes the "acid trigger" that makes virtually every subsequent event in the sequence possible. Reducing acid means less pepsinogen, less pepsin, less secretin, less CCK, less pancreatic enzymes, and less bile.

3. With less acid to feed back and turn down gastrin production, gastrin levels soar. As we discuss below, the excessively high levels of gastrin have been linked to a form of stomach cancer.

4. Since the absorption of many vitamins, minerals, proteins, and amino acids occurs only within a narrow range of pH, disrupting the gastric digestive environment by reducing acidity (raising pH) adversely affects the processing and absorption of many of these nutrients.

5. Consequently, even if we eat an excellent diet, if stomach acid levels are very low, we may be unknowingly partially starving ourselves. Not surprisingly, nutritional deficiencies are a common finding in people with long-standing atrophic gastritis as well as in people taking certain acid-suppressing drugs (see chapter 4.)

Pumping Acid with Gastrin

HCl is secreted by parietal cells, which are located in the gastric mucosa, primarily in the fundus and body of the stomach (see Figure 3-3). This acid is molecularly identical to the HCl that comes in those heavy glass bottles with the glass stoppers in high school chem lab. It is the same stuff as muriatic acid, which has long been used for heavy-duty cleaning and other industrial purposes. It is very strong stuff. During the periods between meals, relatively little acid is secreted, but it is enough to keep the pH of the lumen (or inside cavity) of the stomach between pH 1 and pH 3. However, once food enters the stomach (or even following the sight, smell, taste, or thought of food), acid secretion begins to increase, reaching its maximal rate within about two hours. Acid levels return to their premeal baseline by four to five hours after the beginning of a meal.

The amount of HCl in the stomach at any one time is largely controlled by the hormone gastrin, which is released from G cells located in the stomach lining, or mucosa. As the intragastric pH rises above 3 (less acidic), G cells begin to secrete more gastrin, which triggers parietal cells to start pumping out more HCl into the stomach. The rising acid tide lowers the pH, signaling the G cells to slow their secretion of gastrin, which slows the flow of acid, and so on. In the absence of food, this balanced feedback system keeps the "resting" pH somewhere between 1 and 3 in most people.[3]

Food upsets the balance, because most foods have pHs somewhere around "neutral" (pH 7). So food entering the stomach automatically raises the pH in the surrounding fundus and body, kicking gastrin-HCl secretion into a higher gear. As long as the pH stays above 3, gastrin will continue to stimulate parietal cells to pump acid. As the pH drops back into the 2–3 range, G cells slow their release of gastrin. In addition to the pH stimulus, G-cells also release gastrin in response to certain food constituents, including peptides, amino acids, calcium, as well as certain elements in coffee, wine, and beer.

Gastrin also stimulates acid release indirectly by signaling ECL cells to secrete histamine. The histamine, in turn, binds to H_2 receptors, turning on the acid release pumps.

In addition to its secretory functions, gastrin also controls the muscular actions of the stomach, referred to as *gastric motility*. Muscle contractions propel the stomach contents back and forth, mixing them completely, and at the appropriate time, propelling them out of the stomach and into the duodenum and small intestine. Gastrin reduces stomach motility, which slows gastric emptying.

Inhibiting gastric motility helps the stomach hold and process a large meal. Other factors that influence the rate of gastric emptying include the volume of contents (motility increases as volume increases), pH (lower, pH slows emptying), and composition of the meal (liquids empty faster than solids; fats delay emptying).

The Dangers of Disrupting the Gastrin-Acid Balance

The stomach is very happy as long as the acid-gastrin feedback system hums along smoothly. It starts to act up when the secretion of gastrin, acid, or both goes too far up or too far down for too long.

When acid secretion is too low, the "resting" pH rises higher than the normal gastric pH, 1–3. The elevated pH sends a wake-up call to the G cells, which start spewing out more gastrin to prod the parietal acid pumps to work harder. Acid secretion may appear normal, because the G cells are working a little harder to make up the deficit, but gastrin levels are higher than they should be. Above-normal gastrin secretion is termed *hypergastrinemia*, and it is a potentially serious condition that can lead to gastric adenocarcinoma—a form of stomach cancer.[4] This is discussed in detail in chapter 5.

Hypergastrinemia typically occurs in people with atrophic gastritis (atrophied, thinned, underfunctional or nonfunctional stomach lining) or in those who take powerful acid-blocking drugs for long periods of time. The amount of gastrin in play at any one time is a direct reflection of the current level of stomach acid. Insufficient acid levels (pH greater than 3) in gastric atrophy trigger higher gastrin levels as the body tries to compensate for loss of acidity. Taking a standard 20-mg daily dose of Prilosec typically results in up to a three- to fourfold increase in gastrin levels.[5] In people whose heartburn/GERD fails to respond to the standard dose, long-term treatment with doses as high as 40 or 60 mg has produced gastrin levels as much as tenfold above normal.[6-17]

Why Doesn't the Stomach Digest Itself?

With all that potent acid floating around the stomach, the question inevitably arises, why doesn't the stomach digest itself? How is the thin, delicate lining of the stomach protected while the equally delicate lining of the esophagus is not?

In fact, the protection afforded the stomach lining is as simple as it is effective. It consists primarily of two substances: *mucus* and *bicarbonate*, which are secreted by cells in the epithelial lining (top cell layer) itself.

Mucus is a clear fluid that serves to lubricate and protect delicate epithelial tissue throughout the GI and other respiratory systems. Gastric mucus is not much different from the fluid that runs out of our noses when we have a cold. Consisting largely of water (95 percent) and a small portion of a sugar-protein substance called a glycoprotein (5 percent), it has a slightly gel-like quality that helps it stick to the epithelial lining and serve as a physical buffer against stomach acid and other digestive juices.

Bicarbonate is alkaline and very effective at neutralizing potent acids. Bicarbonate ions are secreted by cells in the lining of the stomach and duodenum in response to contact with acid. Coating the gastric epithelium, along with mucus, they neutralize any acid they come in contact with. So effective is this mucus-bicarbonate barrier that when the pH is 2 (very acidic) in the lumen, or cavity, of the stomach, the pH at the stomach's lining approaches 7, or neutral.

The esophagus is strictly a *transport* organ, not a *digestive* organ. Acid does not belong in the esophagus, because there are no cells in the esophageal lining to secrete protective mucus or bicarbonate. The esophagus is not totally at the mercy of refluxing acid, though. It gets some protection from saliva, which is slightly alkaline. Thus, swallowing saliva not only helps wash refluxing acid out of the esophagus, it also neutralizes it to a certain degree. At the same time, acid in the esophagus triggers a series of wavelike peristaltic contractions designed to send the acid back to the stomach where it belongs.

An intact protective barrier in the stomach is essential to health. Inflammation (gastritis) or ulcers may occur in regions of the stomach where the barrier has been breached. *Like heartburn, ulcers were, for many years, thought to be caused by too much acid. In fact, gastric ulcers often occur in people whose acid levels are low.* It is now widely accepted that most ulcers are initiated by a disruption in the protective barrier, most frequently caused by the bacteria *Helicobacter pylori* but also by certain drugs (e.g., aspirin and other nonsterioidal anti-inflammatory drugs, NSAIDs), which are *exploited* by stomach acid.

Hiatal Hernia

The chest cavity and abdomen are separated by a large sheet of muscle called the *diaphragm*. Above the diaphragm lie the heart and lungs. Below it lie the stomach, pancreas, liver, gallbladder, intestines, and the rest of the digestive organs. The esophagus passes through the diaphragm via an opening called a hiatus. It is not uncommon for a portion of the stomach

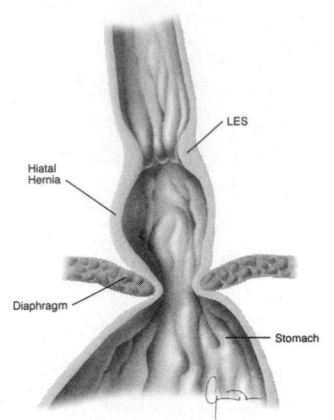

Figure 3-5. Schematic diagram of hiatal hernia.

to protrude though the hiatus into the chest cavity. This condition is known as a *hiatal* (or *hiatus*) *hernia* (see Figure 3-5).

It is estimated that as many as 25 percent of people aged 50 years and older have a hiatal hernia. These hernias are more likely to occur in people who are overweight or pregnant. Normally, the LES aligns with the diaphragm, which helps keep the valve closed except when it is supposed to open following a swallow. However, when there is a hiatal hernia, the LES rises above the diaphragm, which helps weaken the valve and increase the chances of reflux. Also, the acidic gastric juice may accumulate in the herniated portion of the stomach and flow back into the esophagus. Hiatal hernias were once believed to be the primary cause of heartburn. It is known today, though, that they are only one factor. Most hiatal hernias, while troublesome, do not require any special attention. However, large ones can cause serious problems and may require surgery.

CHAPTER 4
Starving in the Midst of Plenty:
How Stomach Acid Levels Affect Nutrient Absorption

Elaine and Tom MacDonald walked into my office, Tom guiding Elaine as unobtrusively as he could. He showed her a chair, and they both sat down.

"As you may have guessed, I'm not seeing as well as I'd like," Elaine began. "My eye doctor tells me it's macular degeneration in both eyes, though the left is worse than the right. I've been taking those vitamins that eye doctors are starting to recommend these days, but they don't seem to be helping at all, and my vision is slowly getting worse."

"We've heard you have a treatment that can help macular degeneration sometimes," Tom said. "We're hoping it's not to late to help Elaine."

"As it is now, I can read an interstate highway sign if I'm standing right in front of it," Elaine said. "And that's with my glasses on. I was a teacher before I retired, and I so miss being able to read my books and newspapers."

"Of course, she can't drive anywhere either," Tom added.

"How's your health otherwise?" I asked.

"As far as I can tell, it's OK. I don't have the energy I'd like, but then I'm sixty-seven, so I guess that's to be expected," Elaine responded.

"No other bothersome symptoms?"

"None that I can think of. "

I asked about her health history, family health history, diet, and exercise. Then we went to an examination room for a physical exam. All appeared OK until we got to her fingers. Her nails bent very easily.

"Excuse me, but your fingernails aren't very strong, are they?"

"They've been that way all my life. Never have been able to grow nice nails like some women do. Mine, they crack, peel, chip . . . I took gallons of gelatin when I was younger, but it never helped. The last few years I've been taking a lot of calcium, it helps a little. They're stronger for awhile, but then bad again. Can't really put it together with anything."

"Do you get cramps in your legs?"

"Yes."

"How often?"

"Oh, two or three times a week, especially at night, but occasionally when I've been doing a lot of walking. But there's nothing unusual about that, is there? Tom gets them, too, and so do some of our friends. We thought it just went with our time of life, like this gray hair." She touched her head.

"You're right, those of us past fifty do get more leg cramps than younger people, but those cramps aren't an inevitable part of aging. They're a correctable malfunction."

I made a few notes. We finished her exam and went back to my office.

"What shall I do first about my eyes?" Elaine asked. "I'm anxious to get started right away."

"First, have your stomach tested . . . "

"My stomach? How will that help my eyes?"

"As we get older, an increasing number of symptoms and health problems need to be approached by checking the stomach and the rest of the digestion first. By the time we're sixty, at least half of us who have symptoms or health problems have problems with digestion and nutrient assimilation. The leg cramps that you and many past-fifty people have are usually a symptom of inadequate digestion and assimilation of calcium, magnesium, potassium, and other minerals."

"In your particular case, it's likely you've had digestion/assimilation problems for years. If we don't patch up these problems as best we can, we won't have as much of a chance to help your eyes, since all the nutrients our eyes need enter our bodies through the digestive tract."

"Maybe that's why these vitamins the eye doctor gave me aren't working?"

"Likely that's part of it, but they don't have all the necessary nutrients, and the few they do contain are in very small quantities."

"Why do you think I've had digestion problems for years? I don't have any digestive symptoms, as far as I can tell."

"Your fingernails. A large majority of women who have cracking, peeling, chipping fingernails also have poor stomach and digestive function."

"Really? You're saying I could have had glamorous fingernails all these years had I only known?"

"Don't know about glamorous, but at least a lot stronger. But getting back to tests . . . along with the stomach test, we need to check further on your digestion through a stool analysis, looking at mineral levels, amino acids, and hormones, particularly testosterone."

"So far, I think I understand checking my digestion and the minerals . . . even these vitamins you say are weak . . . but amino acids? Testosterone?"

"Amino acids are the building blocks of protein. If we hope to rebuild cells and tissues, we need to make sure amino acids are adequate. Yours have a higher probability of being low—"

"Because of poor digestion and assimilation."

"Exactly."

"But what about testosterone?" Tom asked. "What does that have to do with eyes?"

"It's certainly not the most important factor, but vision is so important that we want to cover all the bases right away. Testosterone is the most powerful anabolic steroid that our bodies make naturally. Anabolic steroids do much more than stimulate the growth of muscles. They stimulate repair and regrowth of many damaged body tissues. I've observed that correcting unusually low levels of testosterone can help tissue repair in either sex."

"How long will it take to get the tests done so I can get started?"

"The tests are important, but I recommend you start treatment today or tomorrow, as soon as your tests are turned in. Over the years, I've found that if we give key nutrients intravenously, particularly zinc and selenium, twice weekly, we make much faster progress. We make sure the quantities are safe, of course, but also sufficient to do the job."

"Just zinc and selenium?"

"Those are the most important minerals, but we make sure to back them up with a variety of minerals and other nutrients. And, of course, I'll ask you to start with oral supplementation, too."

"But what about digesting and assimilating them properly?"

"Your stomach test will be completed and the results known today; the remaining tests on your digestion will be completed in just two or three days."

"What about the rest of the tests? Shouldn't we wait for them?" Tom asked.

"We'll adjust or add to what we're doing as soon as they become available, but since we know many of the major items of importance, we can start them right away."

"How often does this work?" Elaine asked.

"Not every time, but definitely more than half the time."

"How long before I know one way or another?"

"In my experience, if we use the IVs, digestive aids, all the oral supplements, and hormones, if necessary, you can see . . . literally . . . results starting in four to six weeks. If there's been no improvement in six to eight weeks, then it's not likely this all will help."

"I hope it works for me. In addition to the IVs, what supplements should I take?"

"Very, very likely the list will start with betaine hydrochloride with pepsin with meals, to replace what your stomach likely isn't doing—secreting acid—and pancreatic enzymes after meals. Together, these should restore a large part of weak digestive function.

"We've already covered zinc and selenium, two of the most important minerals. Vitamin E and taurine are very important, too. Bilberry and ginkgo, herbal medications, contain flavonoids and other substances important to the retina. Vitamin A, copper—"

"Hold on," Elaine said. "I can't remember all of this."

"You don't need to. There are several 'combination formulas' available in natural food stores that contain most or all of these ingredients."

"IVs, digestive aids, a combination formula with the nutrients you've recommended . . . anything else?" Tom asked.

"The tests will tell us if amino acids, testosterone, and possibly other hormones are advisable."

"When I start seeing results, how long will I need to continue having IVs?" Elaine asked. "I certainly can't get those done for years and years."

"You won't need to. Remember, much of the problem is due to poor digestion and assimilation, and you'll be taking care of that so oral supplementation has a better chance to do the job. But just for 'insurance,' when the IVs are discontinued, we'll ask you to use some of the key nutrients dissolved in DMSO, which gets them in through the skin. But don't worry about that now, we'll cover it when the time comes.

"Also, please remember that this treatment doesn't work every time. I've observed it to work in a majority of cases; unfortunately, that's not one-hundred percent."

"At least all these nutrients won't hurt me," Elaine said.

"And we'll pray that Elaine's in that majority," Tom said.

"Please do! That'll help, too."

In four weeks, Elaine's vision started to improve. After eight months of treatment, she reported that instead of just being able to read interstate highway signs, she could read books and newspapers again. She's continued her treatment, and five years later has maintained her vision at that level.*

• • •

Let's say we eat the most highly nutritious diet imaginable, containing just the right amounts of every vitamin, mineral, protein, fiber, and other nutrients. But let's also say we have atrophic gastritis or we take an acid blocker, or both. Thanks to the resulting lack of stomach acid, we may still wind up with serious nutritional deficiencies. The reason can be summed up in one word: "*absorption.*"

The reason we have an esophagus, and a stomach, and intestines, and the rest of the GI system is to digest nutrients of all sorts and then absorb them into our bodies. As we discussed in chapter 3, the processes of digestion and absorption depend on the close coordination of a large number of hormones, enzymes, acids, mucus, and other digestive juices. When working normally, this system is so perfectly tuned that acid, pepsin, gastrin, bicarbonate, and many other substances all get secreted at just the right times in just the right amounts to produce just the right pH to prepare the food for optimal digestion and then absorption of every available nutrient.

The most common thing that goes wrong in the stomach is a loss of acid-producing cells, which is accompanied by a fall off in acid production. This disease, known as *atrophic gastritis* (or *gastric atrophy*), increases with

---

*Reprinted from Dr. Jonathan V. Wright's Nutrition and Healing newsletter, Agora South LLC, Baltimore, Maryland 21201 (410) 223-2611

age, affecting more than 30 percent of people over the age of sixty.[1]

As stomach pH rises (remember, higher pH is more alkaline, lower pH is more acid) in people with atrophic gastritis, the complex and finely tuned digestive and absorptive processes get thrown out of balance. As a result, many amino acids, vitamins, minerals, and other nutrients destined for transport across the intestinal lining and into the bloodstream literally "miss the boat" and wind up exiting the body in the feces.

As if "natural" atrophic gastritis were not bad enough, millions of people today gulp down antacids and powerful acid-suppressing drugs to further squelch the free flow of acid so that only a trickle remains. What is this doing to their nutrient absorption? Decades of scientific research have demonstrated that low stomach acid, whether occurring naturally (i.e., atrophic gastritis) or *iatrogenically* (medicine's euphemism for "caused by the doctor"), should be an important concern because of its potentially destructive effects on the nutritive process. We could be eating the richest, most balanced, most nutritious diet possible, but if our stomach acid secretion is too low, we may be missing out on much of the nourishment ourselves and instead nourishing the bacteria in our septic tanks or municipal sewage treatment plants!

In this chapter, we describe how some key vitamins, minerals, and other nutrients get processed in the stomach to make them available for use in the body. We also show what happens to them—and to us—when the intragastric pH starts to rise.

Iron

Among its numerous vital functions in the body, iron is needed to form hemoglobin, the oxygen-carrying pigment that turns red blood cells red. In the absence of sufficient dietary iron to match that used up by the body, the disease called *iron-deficiency anemia* develops. Chronic anemia means that the body's tissues are starved for oxygen. It can sap muscle strength and drain stamina, leaving us feeling weak and tired. Sometimes anemia is signaled by pale membranes on the inside of the eyelids, and/or pale oral membranes, but often it's discovered only by a blood test.

Although there had been anecdotal reports for decades, the connection between stomach acid and iron deficiency anemia first started getting noticed "scientifically" during the 1930s. In one report, deficient stomach acid, described as either *achlorhydria* (complete absence of stomach acid) or *hypochlorhydria* (mild to severe loss of stomach acid), was found in eleven of thirteen children with anemia. In three of the six children with achlorhydria, and five of the seven with hypochlorhydria, the cause of the anemia was determined to be deficient iron absorption.[2] In another study reported thirty years later, thirty-five of forty-four people (80 percent) with chronic iron-deficiency anemia were found to have below normal acid secretion.[3] Iron-deficiency anemia is a well-known consequence of surgical procedures that remove the regions of the stomach where acid is produced (fundus and body).[4]

Whether or not iron gets absorbed depends to a large degree on the chemical form it takes. In various studies, *ferrous* salts (e.g., ferrous sulfate) and *ferric* salts (e.g., ferric chloride) have often been given to experimental animals or human "guinea pigs" with various levels of stomach pH. They have generally found that the absorption of ferric iron (but not ferrous iron) is closely related to pH; the lower the pH (more acidic), the better the iron gets absorbed. The reason is simple. In order for iron to get absorbed in the duodenum and small intestine, it has to be dissolved in a liquid medium (i.e., stomach juice). Ferric iron has no trouble staying in solution as long as the pH is less than 5. But once the pH gets above 5, as it can in people who have atrophic gastritis and/or who take acid-suppressing drugs, ferric iron starts to fall out of solution—to precipitate—and form an insoluble iron salt. When this iron passes through the duodenum and small intestine, instead of getting absorbed into the bloodstream where it can do some good, it passes through—like an express train through a local station—on its way to the colon and ultimate excretion.

By contrast, ferrous salts remain soluble through a much wider range of pH, extending to neutral (7) or slightly above (alkaline). Thus, the amount of acid in the stomach has little or no effect on the absorption of iron from a ferrous salt.[5]

The type of food the iron comes from also makes a big difference in terms of absorption. A common source of a highly bioavailable source of iron—known as *heme iron*—is meat. Like ferrous chloride, heme iron remains soluble even if the pH rises above 7. If we eat a lot of meat, we absorb lots of iron no matter how much acid our stomachs might be secreting. However, iron that comes from "nonheme" sources, such as grains and vegetables, as well as that which comes from iron "fortification" of some foods, is usually much harder to absorb, for two main reasons. First, it must be released from its fibrous carrier, and second, it must be dissolved.

The secret ingredient in this dual reaction, of course, is HCl. Gastric acid first breaks the chemical bonds that hold the iron molecules, freeing them from the food, and then it converts them from insoluble ferric salts to more soluble ferrous salts. As gastric pH rises, though, absorption of "vegetarian iron" falls. Laboratory research using test-tube procedures have shown that virtually all fiber-bound iron gets absorbed only when the gastric pH is less than 4.0.[6]

A South African study explored the relationship between iron and pH by extracting samples of gastric juice from people who were known to be either normal or iron deficient.[7] After adding the gastric juice samples to pieces of bread containing a known amount of "nonheme" iron, the investigators measured the ability of each sample to extract the iron in the bread and dissolve it. The results were very clear. When the pH of the sample was less than 2, gastric juice had little trouble dissolving the iron. When the pH was higher than 2, though, the ability of gastric juice to solubilize the iron was sharply curtailed.

In the second phase of the study, the researchers gave pieces of iron-fortified bread (now containing a radioactive isotope "tracer" of iron) to the same people, but this time for them to eat. A while later they measured the amount of radioactive iron absorbed by the test subjects' bodies. In this "real life" situation, iron absorption correlated quite well with the ability of each subject's gastric juice to dissolve the iron in the earlier, test-tube phase of the experiment. The better the juice was at dissolving the iron in a test tube, the better the iron was absorbed by the GI tracts of actual living people. Based on those results, the researchers concluded that stomach pH was "the only factor in gastric juice of importance in modifying the absorption of nonheme iron."[7]

Given these results, it comes as no surprise that when supplementary HCl is given to people with anemia and low stomach acid, their iron absorption improves and their anemia disappears. This was demonstrated in a study in which people with anemia and very low stomach acid levels were given iron (ferric chloride) dissolved in water on one day and HCl on another. The mean rate of absorption on "acid days" was

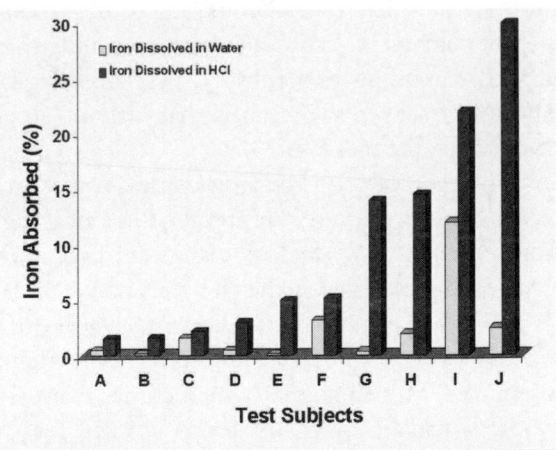

Figure 4-1. Replacing HCl improves iron absorption in people with anemia and low stomach acid levels. Iron (ferric chloride) was dissolved either in water or HCl. On average, more than 300 percent more iron dissolved in acid was absorbed compared with iron dissolved in water. Adapted from PJ Jacobs et al., 1963.

9.2 percent, compared with only 2.2 percent on "water days" (see Figure 4-1).[8]

Why doesn't iron precipitate out of solution once it reaches the duodenum and small intestine, where the environment becomes less acidic than the stomach? The reason is that, while iron remains in solution in the acidic stomach, it combines with certain molecules known as *ligands*, which can help the iron remain dissolved even after the pH rises to 7 and above. Common ligands include ascorbic acid (vitamin C), proteins, amino acids, and sugars. This explains why taking vitamin C with an iron supplement can improve iron absorption. However, in order for these ligands to combine with iron, the iron must first be dissolved in an acidic solution.[9]

Antacids and Iron

By taking neutralizing antacids or acid-suppressing drugs, we may be interfering with normal iron absorption. Swedish researchers found that a liquid neutralizing antacid (similar to Maalox) containing aluminum hydroxide, magnesium hydroxide, and magnesium carbonate significantly reduced the absorption of iron supplements containing either ferrous carbonate, ferrous fumarate, or ferrous sulfate. The absorption of ferrous sulfate was reduced by 38 percent and the fumarate by 31 percent. The ferrous carbonate was completely insoluble when taken with the antacid.[10]

In another study, U.S. researchers compared iron absorption when iron supplements (ferrous sulfate) were taken with either aluminum hydroxide/magnesium hydroxide (e.g., Maalox II, Mylanta), sodium bicarbonate ("bicarb"), or calcium carbonate (e.g., Tums). The results showed that the Maalox II had little or no effect on iron absorption, but the other two antacids profoundly inhibited absorption. Sodium bicarbonate reduced iron absorption by 50 percent, and calcium bicarbonate by 67 percent (see Figure 4-2).[11]

Note that these antacid studies employed *ferrous* salts, which

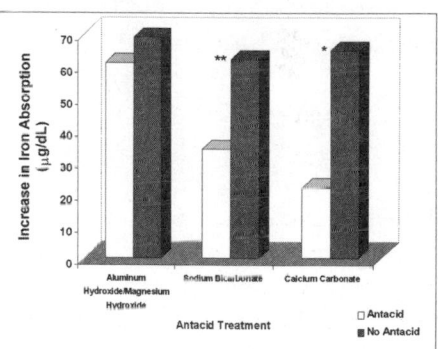

Figure 4-2. Reduction in iron absorption associated with antacid use. Iron levels in plasma were measured two hours after taking an iron supplement (ferrous sulfate) with or without an antacid. Both the antacids tested, sodium bicarbonate and calcium carbonate, sharply reduced iron absorption, while aluminum/magnesium hydroxide had little effect. Adapted from O'Neil-Cutting and Crosby, 1986.

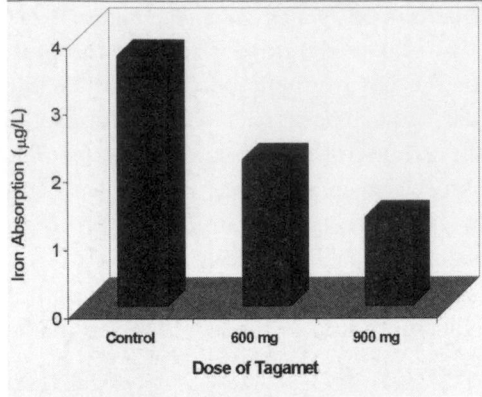

Figure 4-3. Reduction in iron absorption in test subjects taking the acid-suppressing drug Tagamet. As the dose of Tagamet increased, the absorption of iron declined by 42 percent (600 mg) and 65 percent (900 mg).

are commonly used in iron supplements and which are normally easily absorbable, even when pH rises into the alkaline range. Why then did these antacids have such marked effect on iron absorption? It appears that this effect had less to do with pH and more to do with the formation of insoluble salts (e.g., ferric carbonate) by the combination of the antacid with the iron compound.

These experiments do not ask or answer the question, "How does simply reducing stomach acidity affect the absorption of iron from food?" This question was investigated in a study in which normal volunteers ate "test meals" (e.g., hamburger, French fries, vanilla milkshake) containing a known amount of iron after taking the acid-suppressing drug Tagamet. The results showed a highly significant, 28 percent decrease in iron absorption when the subjects took a standard dose of Tagamet (300 mg). Increasing the dose to 600 mg and 900 mg resulted in even greater decreases of 42 percent and 65 percent, respectively (see Figure 4-3).[12]

Calcium

Calcium is an extremely important mineral that the body uses to make bones and teeth strong, among hundreds, if not thousands, of other functions. For example, calcium ions are also essential for many different metabolic and other reactions, including the transmission of nerve impulses in the brain and the contraction and relaxation of muscles, such as those that make the heart beat. Loss of calcium, from either poor nutrition or age-associated causes, can leave bones thin, brittle, and easily broken, a condition known as osteoporosis.

The importance of stomach acid for the absorption of calcium was first noted in the 1960s at a time when high doses of calcium carbonate (e.g., Tums) were one of the principal medical treatments for peptic ulcers. Concerned about the possibility of *excess* calcium absorption, one group of researchers noted that some ulcer patients were barely absorbing any calcium at all—just 2 percent. Looking closer, they found that these people had very little stomach acid; their mean gastric pH was 6.5. However, when they gave one of these people an HCl supplement (betazole hydrochloride), lowering the pH to 1, calcium absorption rose five-fold to 10 percent (see Figure 4-4).[13]

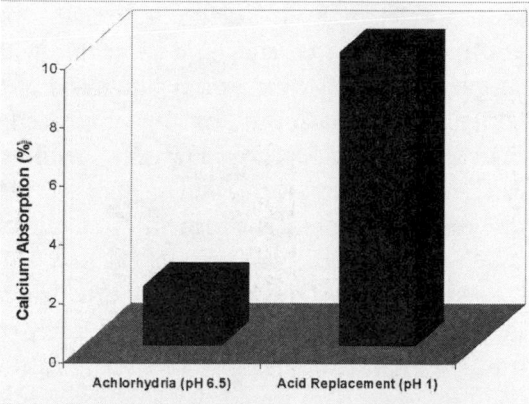

Figure 4-4. Acid replacement improves calcium absorption. Replacement of missing HCl in one achlorhydric patient with betazole HCl improved calcium absorption by a factor of 10. Source: Ivanovich et al., 1967.

Although Tums are no longer the treatment of choice for gastric ulcers, in recent years, calcium "fortification" of foods has become a major obsession among food manufacturers wishing to ride the wave of "calcium awareness" presented in the media. (Calcium is currently one of only a small handful of vitamin or mineral supplements endorsed by the FDA.) Yet, we can consume all the calcium-enriched foods, calcium supplements, and Tums we want and still wind up with a calcium deficiency, if we have low stomach acid due to atrophic gastritis or acid-suppression heartburn "therapy." As with iron, the amount of calcium that gets absorbed depends to a large degree on both the source of the calcium and the pH of the stomach contents. One very common source of calcium, *calcium carbonate*, usually derived from oyster shells or limestone, is often used in calcium supplements and antacids (e.g., Tums). Are these really a good source of calcium? Well, it depends.

Calcium carbonate reacts with HCl to neutralize the acid and form *calcium chloride*, which is a highly soluble salt, that gets easily absorbed in the small intestine shortly after it leaves the stomach—in solution. The problem with calcium carbonate as a source of calcium, though, is that the amount we absorb is a direct function of the amount of acid present in our stomachs. If a person has atrophic gastritis and/or takes an acid-suppressing drug, calcium absorption from calcium carbonate will be markedly curtailed. (A better source of supplemental calcium is *calcium citrate* or *calcium malate* which is more soluble, even when acid secretion is low.)

Other research has confirmed the need for adequate acid secretion to absorb calcium from calcium carbonate, but one study[14] showed that absorption could be enhanced in people with achlorhydria by taking the supplement along with a meal composed of eggs, toast, orange juice, and coffee. The mechanism for this improved absorption may have been demonstrated by Professor Harvey Carroll, who experimentally combined calcium carbonate with orange juice (a rich source of citric acid) and demonstrated significant formation of calcium citrate,[15] noted above as a much more absorbable source of calcium.

As with iron, the absorption of calcium is a twofold process: first, extracting the calcium from its fibrous (vegetarian) carrier, then getting it into solution. Laboratory studies using calcium-containing corn bran and soy hull fibers have found that the upper pH limit for significant calcium absorption was 4.5.[16] Most antacid treatments and acid-blocking drugs are more than capable of raising the gastric pH to 5 or higher. Thus, it would seem likely that using these drugs should reduce calcium absorption. Surprisingly, though, the only study to examine this issue failed to find any effect of Tagamet treatment (which produced a gastric pH of 4.9 to 5.5) on calcium absorption in healthy young test subjects.[17] However, this study has been criticized due to the methodology employed, and its results and conclusion—that Tagamet does not affect calcium absorption—remain doubtful in light of other studies showing that low acid levels inhibit calcium absorption.[18]

Given the importance of calcium absorption for health, one might expect that the pharmaceutical companies that make and market drugs that nearly eliminate acid from the stomach would be interested in finding out what their drugs do to calcium absorption. But alas, aside from the one study mentioned above, no others have ever been published. It's easy to understand why. As long as no one is making a big fuss about nutrient absorption, and no one (i.e., public demand or the FDA) is forcing the pharmaceutical companies to do the relevant studies, they'd rather not know.

Folic Acid

Folic acid (folate) is a B vitamin that, among other uses, is vital for keeping the cardiovascular system healthy by helping to reduce levels of the amino acid homocysteine, and for preventing certain birth defects (e.g., spina bifida). Folate levels tend to decline with advancing age, leading to a rise in homocysteine levels that has been linked to an increased risk of cardiovascular disease. This may partly explain why the risk of cardiovascular disease increases as we age. Adequate folic acid intake (400–800 micrograms/day) easily prevents these problems, but few people ingest enough of the vitamin in their normal diet. To make matters worse, low stomach acid levels, such as those that occur in gastric atrophy, can interfere with folate absorption by raising the pH in the small intestine. When folic acid is given to achlorhydric patients along with some HCl, absorption of the vitamin increases by 54 percent.[19]

However, the issue of folate absorption in chronic low acid states is complicated by the paradoxical fact that elderly people with atrophic gastritis usually have normal or even elevated folate levels in their bloodstreams. How can this be?

It appears that Nature has built in a safety mechanism to prevent folate deficiencies, although this device can be a two-edged sword. As we discuss in chapter 5, low gastric acid secretion results in an overgrowth of bacteria within the confines of the stomach, which are normally nearly sterile. Researchers have found that these hordes of invading bacteria actually produce folate themselves, thus helping to make up the deficiency caused by low acid levels.

While these bacteria may be performing a service in the case of folic acid, bacterial overgrowth is also associated with deficiencies in other nutrients, which the microorganisms actually "steal" from the body and use for themselves. Bacterial overgrowth also raises the risk of bacterial infections leading to discomfort (e.g., diarrhea, flatulence) and even death from serious bacterial diseases (e.g., salmonella, dysentery, cholera). All things being equal, the best way to maintain normal folate levels is to keep the stomach acid flowing, and eat a diet rich in folic acid and/or folic acid supplements rather than relying on abnormal overgrowth of intestinal germs!

How Acid Suppression Affects Folate Absorption

One good way to reduce folate absorption is to take neutralizing antacids or acid-suppressing drugs. A study by researchers from the U.S. Department of Agriculture (USDA) compared folate absorption in thirty normal, healthy men and women aged fifty-five and older, who took either Mylanta II, Tagamet, or Zantac following a meal containing 200 μg of folic acid.[20] Both Tagamet and Zantac significantly raised the intragastric pH from about 1 to 2 before treatment to 5.5 to 6.5 after, respectively. (No posttreatment pH values were reported for the Mylanta II–treated group.) Folate absorption was reduced in all three treatment groups, although the reduction in the Zantac group was not statistically significant (see Figure

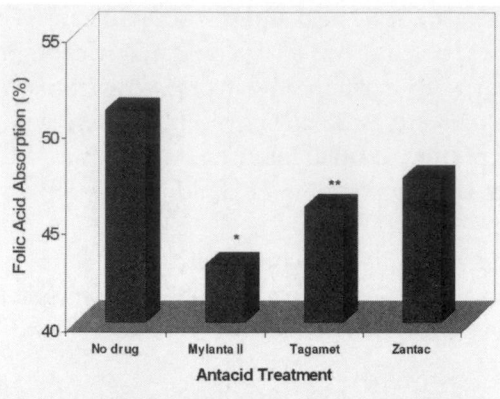

Figure 4-5. Reduction in folic acid absorption associated with neutralizing antacids and acid-suppressing drugs. Healthy test subjects consumed a test meal containing 200 mg of folic acid and took either Mylanta II, Tagamet, or Zantac. P < 0.001. Adapted from Russell et al., 1998.

4-5).[21] The overall reduction in folate absorption was about 16 percent. Although 16 percent less folate is probably not enough to harm an otherwise healthy person, it might adversely affect the health of many other people, including those who take multiple antacids for weeks, months, or years at a time; have serious atrophic gastritis, or eat a diet low in folate content.

Keep in mind that chronically low folate levels are associated with elevated homocysteine levels, which are in turn associated with atherosclerosis and an increased risk of cardiovascular disease. Given these facts, it doesn't seem too far fetched to speculate that chronically low stomach acid could increase the risk of suffering a heart attack or stroke some day. It's highly doubtful that any pharmaceutical company is doing serious research to explore that possibility.

Vitamin B₁₂

We need vitamin B_{12} (cobalamin) for normal nerve activity and brain function. Among its other important uses, vitamin B_{12}, in combination with folate and vitamin B_6, helps keep homocysteine levels under control. Low levels of vitamin B_{12} can leave us feeling dull, tired, and depressed. In children, low stomach acidity along with poor absorption of vitamin B_{12} has been linked to the occurrence of asthma (see chapter 6.)

Vitamin B_{12} typically enters the body bound to food proteins, almost exclusively animal-derived foods, including meat, eggs, and dairy products. In order for us to absorb vitamin B_{12}, the vitamin molecules must first be separated from this protein with the help of stomach acid and pepsin. Once free, vitamin B_{12} quickly combines with another kind of protein binder, which originates in the salivary glands, stomach, liver, pancreas, and other GI organs. As the re-bound vitamin B_{12} enters the small intestine (where the pH has risen to near neutral), enzymes from the pancreas (pancreatic proteases) break the vitamin free again so it can now combine with a substance with the rather prosaic name *intrinsic factor.*

Intrinsic factor is secreted by parietal cells in the stomach, the same cells that produce and release HCl. The vitamin B_{12}-intrinsic factor complex then travels almost the entire length of the small intestine to the terminal ileum. Here it binds to specific receptors and is quickly absorbed into the bloodstream.[22]

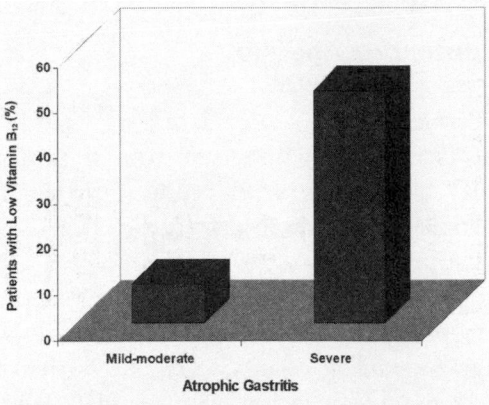

Figure 4-6. Severe atrophic gastritis reduces vitamin B_{12} absorption. Vitamin B_{12} levels were measured in elderly people with low stomach acid pepsin, and intrinsic factor due to atrophic gastritis. Source: Krasinski, 1986

Looking back on this sequence of events, it's easy to see how an acid deficiency can disrupt vitamin B_{12} absorption. If vitamin B_{12} does not get dissociated from its food protein binder in the stomach by HCl and pepsin, the chain is broken almost before it begins, and none of the other subsequent events can occur.

Vitamin B_{12} deficiencies tend to occur most often in elderly people, especially those who have atrophic gastritis (remember this occurs frequently when we're older). When gastric acid secretion is low in older people, pepsin production is also reduced. Moreover, the loss of parietal cells in atrophic gastritis also means that less intrinsic factor is produced. Thus, when a piece of meat or fish is eaten, the vitamin B_{12} stays locked onto its protein carrier and never gets absorbed.

In one study, 32 percent of a group of 359 people aged sixty to ninety-nine years was found to have atrophic gastritis. Vitamin B_{12} levels in participants' bodies were closely related to the extent of their disease. In those with mild to moderate gastritis, only 8.5 percent had a vitamin B_{12} deficiency. However, when atrophic gastritis was severe, more than 50 percent had low vitamin B_{12} (see Figure 4-6).[23]

Low stomach acid also affects vitamin B_{12} absorption indirectly by encouraging bacterial overgrowth in the stomach. While these bacteria have been known to return the favor by producing more folate and vitamin B_6, they are not so forthcoming with vitamin B_{12}. In fact, they may steal it away for themselves. Some use it to nourish their own cells, while others simply inactivate it so it can't do anyone any good.

Pernicious Anemia

"Pernicious" anemia is a serious vitamin B_{12} deficiency that can occur in people with severe atrophic gastritis, resulting in the loss of HCl, pepsin, and, especially, intrinsic factor. It gets its name because people commonly died from it in the days before the discovery of vitamin B_{12}.

What distinguishes pernicious anemia from garden-variety atrophic gastritis is its severity. In severe pernicious anemia, the damage to parietal cells is so extensive that they lose their ability to secrete intrinsic factor as well as HCl. Without intrinsic factor, even if there were enough acid, vitamin B_{12} could never get absorbed down in the southern end of the small intestine. If it misses this stop along the digestion express, the next stop is the colon and excretion. Pernicious anemia this bad can be treated only with vitamin B_{12} injections, which work very well. (They don't cure the basic problem, which is complete failure of stomach function, but they do make up the deficit of vitamin B_{12}.) Pernicious anemia can also occur when atrophic gastritis is less extensive, due to the relative lack of acid and pepsin, the first step in the digestion-absorption of vitamin B_{12}. People with the milder forms of pernicious anemia may also benefit from B_{12} injections, but they should first try HCl/pepsin supplementation to restore their stomach acid levels.

How Acid-Blocking Drugs Affect Vitamin B_{12} Absorption

By suppressing the secretion of HCl, pepsin, and intrinsic factor, acid-suppressing drugs are quite capable of causing a vitamin B_{12} deficiency. In one study, administration of Tagamet to twelve duodenal ulcer patients resulted in significant malabsorption of protein-bound vitamin B_{12}. Interestingly, crystalline vitamin B_{12}, which is not bound to protein, was easily absorbed. This suggests that malabsorption in this case occurs due to the lack of sufficient acid and pepsin to release the vitamin B_{12} from its protein carrier.[24]

Several studies show that Prilosec treatment can interfere with vitamin B_{12} absorption. A group of USDA researchers from Tufts University compared the absorption of protein-bound vitamin B_{12} in a group of elderly people with normal stomach acid, a group with

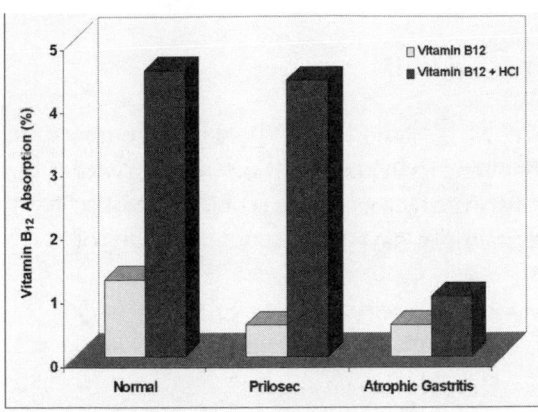

Figure 4-7. Prilosec inhibits vitamin B_{12} absorption; HCl restores it. Elderly test subjects consumed protein-bound vitamin B_{12}. Those taking Prilosec and those with atrophic gastritis absorbed significantly less vitamin than normal controls. Administration of vitamin B_{12} + HCl resulted in a substantial improvement in absorption in both the normal and Prilosec groups. Adapted from JR Saltzman et al., 1994.

low acid due to atrophic gastritis, and a group taking Prilosec.[25] They found that significantly less B_{12} was absorbed by the Prilosec and atrophic gastritis groups, compared with the group with normal stomach acid (see Figure 4-7).[26] In other words, Prilosec produces a state of functional atrophic gastritis in which vitamin B_{12} absorption is inhibited. Low acid and pepsin levels in both conditions, inhibited the release of the protein-bound vitamin. However, when the B_{12} was taken with a small amount of dilute HCl, absorption shot up dramatically in both the normal control and Prilosec groups. The small response to HCl the atrophic gastritis group may have been due to the lack of intrinsic factor or pepsin in these individuals.

In another study, Prilosec (20 or 40 mg) was tested in a group of ten healthy men aged twenty-two to fifty-five years. Stomach acid levels declined to near-zero, paralleling a dramatic decline in vitamin B_{12} absorption.[27]

These were short-term studies, but what happens when people take Prilosec and similar drugs daily for months or years at a time? There is little long-term data evaluating vitamin B_{12} levels in people taking these drugs. However, one review found that, despite the inhibition of absorption, levels tend to stay fairly normal for the first three to four years of use, perhaps due to large stores of the vitamin. After four years of treatment, though, vitamin B_{12} levels do begin to decline.[28] We should also point out again that most of these studies were conducted in *healthy* men and women. When we start out with low vitamin B_{12} levels due to atrophic gastritis or poor diet, the additional decrease superimposed by Prilosec or other drugs may be just enough to tip the balance into serious vitamin malnutrition.

Reversing a Vitamin B$_{12}$ Deficiency

It is possible to improve vitamin B$_{12}$ absorption in people with low stomach acid. In one study, five people with hypochlorhydria and a vitamin B$_{12}$ deficiency were treated with supplements of HCl, pepsin, intrinsic factor, or some combination of these—simply replacing what was missing. In four out of five, B$_{12}$ absorption was significantly improved.[29]

Zinc

The mineral zinc takes part in many metabolic processes related to keeping cell membranes stable, forming new bone, immune defense, night vision, and tissue growth. Only three studies have evaluated the relationship between gastric pH and absorption of dietary zinc. Of these, two suggest that stomach acid is necessary, while the third found little or no connection. The negative finding came from a study that has been criticized because of a variety of methodological errors that bring the results into serious question.[30]

In a much better controlled trial, Tagamet treatment reduced zinc absorption by about 50 percent.[31] Another study found that Pepcid, which raised the intragastric pH to over 5, had the same effect. The researchers

Does Antacid Use Cause Blindness?

Macular degeneration is the leading cause of irreversible vision loss in the United States associated with advancing age. According to a recent report from the ongoing Age-Related Eye Disease Study (AREDS), it appears that one of the most important risk factors for a subgroup of individuals with "dry" macular degeneration (those characterized by "geographic atrophy") is the use of antacids.

Exactly how antacid use may lead to macular degeneration is uncertain, but it is known that regular antacid use produces maldigestion/malabsorption of zinc and other nutrients just as age-related hypochlorhydria/atrophic gastritis does. Other studies have linked low levels of zinc to the development of macular degeneration.

Thus, by inhibiting the absorption of zinc, long-term use of antacids may lead to macular degeneration and loss of vision.

Source: Age-Related Eye Disease Study Group. Risk factors associated with age-related macular degeneration, *Ophthalmology*. 2000: 107: 2224–2232.

also found that zinc sulfate is better absorbed at high pH than zinc oxide.[32] While this study implies that zinc sulfate is preferable to zinc oxide as a supplement for individuals who have atrophic gastritis or take acid-suppressing drugs, fifteen years of clinical experience based on the known biochemistry of zinc absorption in humans has shown that the best-absorbed form of supplemental zinc is zinc *picolinate*.

Other Nutrients

Like folate, vitamin B_6 absorption normally requires an acid pH in the stomach. Nevertheless, vitamin B_6 deficiencies are uncommon in elderly people with atrophic gastritis. Again it appears that bacterial overgrowth may be making up the difference. There has been very limited systematic research on the absorption of other nutrients, but there is good reason to believe that low acid levels might also affect levels of vitamin A and vitamin E, thiamin (vitamin B_1), riboflavin (vitamin B_2), and niacin (vitamin B_3). Theoretically, the absorption of any nutrient that is bound to protein (as well as proteins themselves; see below) will be inhibited.[33]

How Low Stomach Acid May Cause Depression

Mention this possibility to most conventional, pharmaceutically oriented physicians and psychiatrists, and they'll probably laugh in your face and tell you you've been reading too many of those "alternative medicine" books. "Just hand me the Prozac, if you please." But the following case is only one (although certainly the most colorful) of literally hundreds I've encountered. *

"I'm seventy-six this year, and my wife Theresa here thinks I'm losing it," said Vincent Parnelli. "I was just passing it off, but now I think she's right. Last week, I drove off and left the boat at the launch for the second time in a month . . . with the dog in it, too. Had the fish in the car, don't know how I thought I caught 'em. Had to drive all the way back to get the boat and the dog . . . "

Theresa reached over to pat his arm. "You're not 'losing it,' dear. You've just been a little more absent-minded these last couple of years."

"Theresa's always putting a good face on things," he said, smiling at her. "But if I can't even remember the boat and the dog, 'losing it' is more accurate. After I did that, I decided to have a good look at how I'm doing.

---

*Reprinted from Dr. Jonathan V. Wright's Nutrition & Healing newsletter, Agora South LLC, Baltimore, Maryland, 21201 (410)-223-2611.

Theresa's been trying to get me to come in here for the last five years, and here I am."

I made a note. "Besides your memory, have you noticed anything else about your health that doesn't seem right?"

"I asked Theresa to come along so she could tell you what she's seeing. Like I said, I've been passing things off, probably too much." He turned to his wife.

"Well . . . ," she hesitated. "Vinnie's been more forgetful for several years now. I mean, we all are now and again, but it's been more than that. I've been finding a lot more socks in the refrigerator, car keys in the laundry, unmailed letters in the car, things like that. To begin with, I just took care of it, but I stopped, because I wanted him to notice, too. When he didn't, I was surprised, so I started pointing things out . . . but until he forgot the boat and dog twice, it didn't make any difference."

"Anything else?"

She looked at her husband. "Vinnie, I'm not being critical, it's because the doctor asked . . . "

This time, he reached over and touched her arm. "It's OK, I want you to tell the doctor everything, I'd probably forget most of it anyway . . . "

"That's another thing, doctor, Vinnie's just been more 'down' the last two or three years. I wouldn't call it depressed exactly. He's not just sitting around staring at the wall or anything, but he's not smiling or laughing the way he has in the past."

"With the politicians we got now, it's enough to depress anyone," Mr. Parnelli said.

"It's more than just politicians. You could even laugh at Roosevelt, Vinnie." She turned to me and smiled. "We've been married a long time."

"Roosevelt, that fascist, totally violated our Constitution . . . but when I really think about it, Theresa's right, I haven't seen as much that's seemed very funny in the last few years. Maybe it's because I'm not sleeping as well as I did when I was younger."

"That too, doctor," Mrs. Parnelli said. "I was reading about depression, just in case, you know, and it said that insomnia and sleeplessness are 'classic symptoms' of depression. Is that true?"

"Depends on your point of view. Depression, insomnia, and forgetfulness could all be symptoms of something else, too," I answered. "I'll explain later on. Any other symptoms or things you've noticed?"

"Let's see," Mrs. Parnelli said. "More forgetful, depressed, not sleeping well . . . and maybe tiring more easily than usual. What do you think, Vinnie?"

"I was just blaming it on being older, I am seventy-six, but Theresa reminded me about my father. He was zipping around doing things until he was over ninety. Especially when I try to work hard, chopping wood or whatever, I get tired out and my muscles just physically get more tired. Like I said, I just put it down to age and not sleeping so good, but with this forgetful thing . . . "

We finished Mr. Parnelli's health history, and went to the examination room. Everything appeared relatively OK until we got to checking his stomach and abdomen.

"Quite a bit of gassiness," I remarked.

"That's been with me for years. Most of my friends, too. Sometimes we even call ourselves the 'gassy grandpas.' Could be worse. A few years before I retired I had a bad stretch of heartburn. Doctor told me no ulcer, just take antacids, it'd pass, and it did."

"With this, your symptoms are forming a fairly typical pattern."

Mr. Parnelli sat up abruptly. "What's a lot of belching and gas got to do with forgetting the boat and the dog?" he demanded.

"Now, Vinnie, let the doctor finish, I'm sure he'll tell us," Mrs. Parnelli soothed. Mr. Parnelli looked doubtful, but lay back down, and we finished his exam.

"So what disease are you finding in whatever pattern you're talking about?" Mr. Parnelli asked. He put his shirt on and sat down, arms crossed.

"No disease, just a frequently occurring pattern of wear-and-tear," I replied.

"Wear and tear? Is that just a polite way of telling me I'm just getting older like I thought, nothing I can do?"

"We're all getting older, but if we pay attention, there's a lot we can do to stay healthy at the same time. Please remember, what I'm going to explain is just a theory until we do some tests and try some treatments, but this same pattern happens to so many of us . . . "

"Gas, belching, and forgetting the dog making a pattern. Wait'll I tell this to Bill . . . "

"Vinnie . . . "

"OK, Theresa, I'll be good and listen."

"As we get older," I explained, "many of us lose digestive capacity, some of us sooner than others. By age sixty, at least half of us have significant digestive slowdown. Usually, our stomachs aren't making as much acid and pepsin as when we were younger, so our food, especially the protein, isn't as well-digested as it might be. And inefficient digestion is very often accompanied by considerable gas. It's very likely that the 'stretch of heartburn' and increasing gas you had before you retired was a signal of progressive stomach failure."

"So if my stomach was making less acid and pepsin than necessary, why did the doctor tell me to take antacids?"

I sighed. "Habit, lack of understanding, inadequate testing . . . really hard to say. But when we carefully test people over age forty who're having heartburn, indigestion, and gas, over 90 percent of the time we find inadequate acid (and presumably pepsin) production by the stomach. Hydrochloric acid and pepsin supplementation relieves the symptoms, further proving the point. That's likely part of what you'll need . . . but let's get back to forgetting the dog.

"Hydrochloric acid and pepsin are what the stomach uses to digest protein. The ultimate products of protein digestion are called amino acids and short chains of amino acids are called 'peptides.' When we test people who have seriously inadequate stomach function, or who've had inadequate stomach function for a long time, we usually find a pattern of lower than average to much lower than average amino acids in the bloodstream. Now, most neurotransmitters are made from amino acids—"

"Neurotransmitters?"

"You remember, Vinnie, I was telling you neurotransmitters are the little molecules the brain cells use for sending messages to each other?" Mrs. Parnelli said. "So if Vinnie's stomach isn't working right, he might not have been digesting enough protein into amino acids for his brain to use to make enough neurotransmitters, so he might get forgetful?"

"Exactly. It could also account for a lot of his sleeplessness and insomnia. Those very often get a lot better when we get people on the right combination of amino acids."

"Isn't muscle made out of amino acids, too?" Mrs. Parnelli asked.

"All proteins are, and muscle is mostly protein."

"So if my stomach doesn't work right, and I'm not getting enough amino acids, then my muscles might get weak, too?" Mr. Parnelli leaned forward, uncrossed his arms, and looked much more interested. "Let's see . . . gas, belching, poor digestion, low amino acids, weak muscles, low neurotransmitters, sleeplessness, insomnia, depression . . . and forgetting the boat and dog. Damn! It all makes sense after all!"

I smiled. "One of the common patterns as we get older, if we're not careful. There are a few more details, too. If the digestion isn't working well, injections of vitamin B_{12} and other B vitamins can be very helpful for the function of the brain and nervous system, and can be especially helpful against fatigue. Over the years, many people with poor stomach function have told me that intravenous injections of essential minerals are very helpful in restoring strength, stamina, and endurance.

"Also, the large majority of us at age seventy-six are quite low on the hormone DHEA, and many of us men are low in testosterone. Supplementing with small quantities of one or both of these hormones in identical-to-natural form can be very useful, even reinvigorating, and can help to rebuild healthy tissue all around the body. Most people notice improvement in mental function, too."

"So when do I get started on all this stuff?"

"Remember, this is all just theory until we get the right tests done. But given the overall pattern, tests will probably show that hydrochloric acid-pepsin replacement, amino acids, B_{12} injections, essential minerals, DHEA, and possibly testosterone will be the items recommended."

"So I may not be 'losing it.' I'm just low on things that belong in my body anyway. It's more like patching and repairing an old house than treating some disease."

"Right."

Mr. and Mrs. Parnelli began to get up, but she sat down with another question. "Aren't there some vitamins and herbs that can help memory and depression, too, doctor?"

"Sure. Ginkgo, acetyl-L-carnitine, and phosphatidylserine all have impressive studies done showing their ability to improve memory and depression, especially when we're older. Let's wait to see how Mr. Parnelli does on the 'home repair' items first, and then consider using one or more of those."

As expected, Mr. Parnelli's tests disclosed weak digestive function, low amino acids, many low minerals, and low DHEA. With the help of the appropriate amino acids, vitamin B_{12} injections (with other B vitamins), minerals, DHEA, and digestive correction, his memory, low-grade depression and other symptoms were much improved within eight months. At that point we added in ginkgo both to try to sharpen memory further, as well as for its action in improving small blood vessel circulation and erectile function. One year later, Mrs. Parnelli told me there had been no more socks in the refrigerator, only "the occasional memory lapse like the rest of us," and Vinnie hadn't forgotten the boat or the dog since.

• • •

While the evidence is largely "anecdotal" and circumstantial at this point, it is at least theoretically possible that having advanced atrophic gastritis or taking acid-suppressing or other drugs daily for months or years at a time could leave a person feeling clinically depressed. The immediate reason is a lack of absorbtion of adequate amounts of the essential amino acids

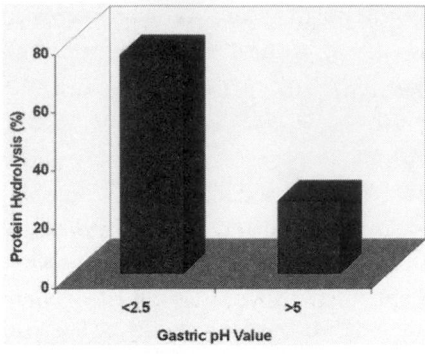

Figure 4-8. Protein digestion (hydrolysis) occurs best when the pH is less than 2.5. The results of this study show that at normal gastric pH (less than 2.5), 75 percent of protein is hydrolyzed, compared with only 25 percent when the pH is high (greater than 5). Adapted from Maltby, 1934.

tryptophan and *phenylalanine*, and the "nonessential" but important amino acid *tyrosine*, and very likely others. The body uses these three amino acids for the production of the neurotransmitters *serotonin* and *norepinephrine* (aka, *noradrenaline*).

Deficiencies in these neurotransmitters are closely associated with depression and other emotional disorders. Drugs like Prozac, Zoloft, Serzone, and others are used to relieve depression because they raise the levels of these neurotransmitters. The amino acids themselves are derived from dietary proteins that are broken apart by the actions of HCl and pepsin in the stomach.

HCl, Pepsin, and Protein Digestion

Protein is digested (*hydrolyzed*) in the stomach to produce amino acids and peptides (two or more amino acids linked together) by the actions of pepsin. This action occurs best when the pH is between 1 and 2. As the gastric pH climbs, the rate of hydrolysis declines.[34] As shown in Figure 4-8, when the gastric pH is less than 2.5 (within the normal range), 75 percent of protein (beef) is hydrolyzed, compared with only 25 percent when the pH is high (greater than 5). Acid-suppressing drugs typically raise the intragastric pH to 5 or higher.

Normal digestion of protein results in the release of essential amino acids, including phenylalanine, tryptophan, valine, and leucine, as well as "nonessential" but important amino acids such as tyrosine and arginine. There is little direct evidence that hypochlorhydria or achlorhydria, whether due to atrophic gastritis or acid-suppressing drugs, inhibits the absorption of essential amino acids. However, there is considerable circumstantial evidence. In one study, people who had had part of their stomachs surgically removed (resulting in less acid secretion), absorbed less protein than a control group with normal stomachs.[35]

Bacterial overgrowth due to chronically low acid levels can also get in the way of normal amino acid absorption. As we noted earlier with vitamin B$_{12}$, some bacteria may hijack the amino acids for their own use, possibly producing toxic byproducts in the process.[36-37]

During the early years of the twentieth century, there were isolated reports that certain products of bacterial metabolism of amino acids could cause a syndrome that resembled what may now be diagnosed as clinical depression. Symptoms included excessive fatigue, reduced ability to concentrate, and insomnia (in people), and somnolence and lack of interest in the external environment (in monkeys).[38]

A more likely connection, as we mentioned above, may be the deficit in at least two neurotransmitters, serotonin and norepinephrine, and their amino acid precursors, tryptophan, phenylalanine, and tyrosine. Numerous reports have confirmed that a large reduction in plasma tryptophan levels can result in depression, especially if the individual is prone to depression due to genetic makeup or family history.[39-45]

Can low stomach acid make us depressed? Although I've found this to be true for many individuals, there are no "controlled studies," so "scientifically" speaking, at this point, the possibility remains nothing more than an intriguing hypothesis.[46] However, should it be borne out by systematic research, it may mean that, for some people at least, treatment for their depression may be as simple as taking HCl supplements, accompanied by amino acids and other "missing" nutrients.

The subject of low stomach acid, amino acids, neurotransmitters and depression is so important that we've included a separate discussion in appendix I.

For Women, Low Stomach Acid Often Causes "Lousy" Fingernails or Hair Loss

In a way, women with low stomach acid are often "lucky" to develop one of two "signs" that men with the same problem rarely encounter: cracking, chipping, peeling, and "layering" fingernails, or overall (not localized) head hair loss. (It's rare to have both poor-quality fingernails and hair loss occur in the same woman.)

Did we say "lucky"? Rapidly thinning hair, or nails only a cosmetologist could love? Lucky, because women with these problems *know* something's the matter and sometimes are also lucky enough to find nutritionally oriented physicians who will help these symptoms to diagnose and correct or compensate for the underlying cause: poor stomach function. "Patching up" the stomach problem helps not only the hair loss and the "lousy" fingernails, but the entire body's nutrition as well!

We men aren't "lucky" enough to develop these telltale symptoms, so we continue to suffer the consequences of poor stomach function.

Why High Fiber and Low Stomach Acid Don't Mix

Dietary fiber includes many different substances found in plant cell walls. For years, we have been told (and rightfully so) to eat more fiber for a variety of preventive and therapeutic purposes. Dietary fiber appears to become even more important as we age, since it may be involved not only in promoting healthy bowel activity, but also in preventing colon cancer and cardiovascular disease by helping to reduce cholesterol levels. Thus, elderly people, in particular, are encouraged to eat foods containing lots of fiber.

But fiber also has a little-known dark side as far as nutrition is concerned. Fiber can bind with nutrients and actually remove them from the body before they have chance to get absorbed. This is especially likely to occur as that old gastric pH starts to rise, as it often does with advancing age or as a result of taking acid-suppressing drugs, or, increasingly, both. By now you know where this is going: Eating a high-fiber diet on a low-acid stomach drives many of these valuable nutrients from the GI system directly into that municipal sewage treatment plant.

Here's how it works in simplified way: Both fiber itself and a constituent called *phytic acid* or *phytate*, are extremely effective at "locking onto" dietary minerals. Phytic acid, which comes from many grains, cereals, and seeds, combines with numerous minerals, including zinc, copper, nickel, manganese, iron, and calcium.

The solubility of these mineral-phytate complexes depends on a complex interaction among a number of factors, including the pH value and the specific mineral(s) involved, among others. In general, mineral-phytate complexes are soluble—and therefore, absorbable—only at low pH (usually less than 3). Test-tube studies, for example, show that zinc and copper phytates start to drop out of solution when the pH gets into the 3 to 4.5 range, and solubility continues to decline as the pH rises. The same thing happens with iron, zinc, copper, and the others, although the pH levels may vary. It also happens with protein, which requires acid and pepsin for digestion.

And just to complicate matters, if there's enough calcium or magnesium present, as they precipitate out of solution, they take some of the other minerals out with them, thus magnifying the loss.[47]

The main reason this nutrient theft doesn't go on all the time is that the normally low gastric pH prevents it by keeping the various mineral-phytate/fiber complexes in solution. However, when the pH starts to rise above 3 to 4, 5, 6, or 7, the minerals begin to precipitate out in the form of insoluble, unabsorbable, and, therefore, *unusable* compounds.

What does this mean for us fiber eaters? It means that if we do all the right things—eat a high-fiber, low-meat diet and maybe throw in some extra calcium (for strong bones)—but have atrophic gastritis or take an acid-blocking drug, or both, we may be starving ourselves of numerous vital nutrients.

The leading scientific voice warning about this potential loss of nutrients has been Elaine T. Champagne, PhD, a researcher with the USDA.[48–50] She argues that the incomplete digestion of protein-mineral-phytate complexes, combined with the incomplete digestion of protein due to inadequate pepsin activity, could be "the most important consequences of raised stomach pH values on mineral nutriture from high-fiber foods." Dr. Champagne warns that elderly people who have elevated stomach pH values and who regularly consume diets that are high in fiber and phytate and low in animal protein "may be at risk of suffering from mineral impairment."[37] Of course, the risk of excess dietary mineral loss is similar every time we take Prilosec, Tagamet, Zantac, Tums, Rolaids, or other acid-blocking/antacid treatment and then eat meals containing dietary fiber.

Research and Clinical Observation

So far, we've written about the clinical research that exists concerning nutrient absorption and naturally occurring or drug-induced low levels of stomach acid. We've noted research concerning iron, calcium, folate, vitamin B_{12}, zinc, and amino acids. We've also mentioned the lessening of nutrient absorption brought about by the combination of low stomach acidity and dietary fiber. But what about all the other nutrients: carotenoids; other B vitamins; vitamins A, C, D, E, K; essential fatty acids; flavonoids; magnesium; copper; chromium; selenium; manganese; biotin; and many others?

Recall that in chapter 3, we described the "digestive cascade," the series of events triggered by fully acidified meals. This "cascade" includes acid-induced hormone release triggering the secretion of bile and pancreatic enzymes. Without the "acid trigger," the rest of the "cascade" doesn't work as well either, and the secretion of bicarbonate and enzymes (trypsin, chymotrypsin, amylase, lipase, elastase, protease, and others) by the pancreas and bile and bile salts by the gallbladder aren't stimulated properly. Absorption of many of the other nutrients noted above can be impaired, even though stomach acid and pepsin may not be directly responsible for their digestion and absorption. In a way, then, normal stomach function is like the first domino in a row: If it doesn't fall as it should, the rest won't either.

In more than thirty years of medical practice, twenty-eight of them nutritionally oriented, I've observed improvement in the absorption of nearly every nutrient when poor stomach function is improved. While it's true that the most frequently affected nutrients include all of the essential minerals except sodium and potassium, and all of the essential amino acids, any one or any combination of the other nutrients can also be involved.

What's presented in this chapter is most of the research that could be found through extensive library and online searching. So where's the research on all the other nutrients? The sad fact is that it hasn't been done yet, even though this is said to be "the most modern scientific era." It's not likely that patent medicine (pharmaceutical) companies with a financial interest in acid blockers or antacids will fund studies on the adverse effects of their money-making drugs and treatments, especially if the adverse effects escape immediate notice. Government grants and the large majority of foundation grants are usually motivated by what's trendy and popular in mainstream medicine. So the money for "hard" research usually isn't there.

All of the problems associated with low stomach acid (of whatever cause) were apparent within my first ten years of medical practice. But since much of the "hard research" hadn't been done, I thought it best to wait for many more years of clinical observation before joining Dr. Lenard in writing this book.

CHAPTER 5
How Low Stomach Acid Can Make You Sick:
The Bacteria-Cancer Connection

We try not to think about it, but the mouth, esophagus, and intestines are virtual bacterial cities, containing more than four-hundred different species of microscopic bugs.[1] But a healthy stomach, which lies directly between the esophagus and the beginning of the intestines, is normally an oasis of sterility, or near sterility. This microbe-free buffer zone exists because of one simple fact: *stomach acid kills bacteria*. "The low pH of the intragastric environment constitutes one of the major non-specific defense mechanisms of the body," wrote one researcher.[2]

The gastric acid barrier guards two gateways simultaneously. Most swallowed or inhaled bacteria play no role in digestion and would constitute an unwelcome alien presence amidst the flourishing *natural* microbial ecology that is essential for digestion in the intestines. Thus, stomach acid intercepts bacteria that enter through the gateway of the nose and mouth and kills them before they can pass into the intestine. By the same token, intestinal bugs have no business farther north, where they can only cause trouble. The acid barrier (a term taken directly from medical textbooks) keeps these bacteria from migrating up through the duodenum and pylorus and putting down roots in the stomach lining.

Although some bacteria can usually be found in a healthy stomach, the vast majority turn out to be recent arrivals. When the pH is 3 or lower, the normal between-meal "resting" level, bacteria don't last more than fifteen minutes (perhaps a little longer if the pH gets up to 4). If we were to completely stop swallowing for fifteen minutes or more, our stomachs would rapidly revert to their naturally sterile or near-sterile state.

As the pH rises to 5 or more, though, many bacterial species avoid the acid treatment and begin to thrive. Without regular acid baths to drive them out, the stomach can become a quite hospitable locale for bacterial colonization. It's dark, it's warm, it's moist, and it's often full of nutrients.[3] Acid-suppressing drugs routinely drive the intragastric pH over 5. Fortunately, most of the bacteria we ingest won't kill us, at least not right away. But some of them will. People who have a gastric pH high enough to promote bacterial growth may be vulnerable to serious bacterial infections such as *Salmonella*, *cholera*, *dysentery*, *typhoid*, and *tuberculosis*,[2] not to mention garden-variety heartburn, diarrhea, constipation, bloating, flatulence, or other common symptoms of *dyspepsia* ("upset stomach").

The evidence is unmistakable. The risk of Salmonella infection is more than threefold in people who have had stomach surgery that inhibits acid secretion, and it rises in direct proportion to the degree that the operation reduces acid-secreting capacity.[4] In a 1970 cholera outbreak in Israel, one-fourth of the twenty-five people who came down with the disease had had prior stomach surgery. Sixteen of the patients had no free stomach acid at all and a mean pH of 6.4. Those people with the least stomach acid (achlorhydria) had the most severe cholera.[5]

In a study of thirty-seven Bangladeshis with cholera, sixteen had deficient stomach acid. When researchers sampled gastric juice from these sixteen people and put these samples into test-tubes with the cholera-causing bacteria, *V. cholerae,* they failed to kill the bug.[6]

In fact, though, *V. cholerae* is exceptionally vulnerable to a low pH.[7] Thus, when the stomach pH is normal (i.e., 3 or less), the risk of developing cholera or any other infectious intestinal disease, even if we happen to drink some tainted water, is much lower. As noted above, the concept of the "acid barrier to gastrointestinal disease" has been firmly established in medical textbooks for many, many decades.

Much that we have said about cholera is also true of Salmonella, typhoid, and nearly all bugs that might infect our intestines. The "acid barrier" isn't 100 percent effective (even children and teenagers with "maximum-strength" stomach acid can get intestinal infections), but it definitely lowers our risk of gastroenteric infection. Elderly people, who are more likely to have low stomach acid due to decades of progressing atrophic gastritis, have been found to be particularly prone to Salmonella infection.[8]

Anti-acid Drugs Can Make Us Vulnerable to Infection

One reason diseases like Salmonella, cholera, typhoid, and dysentery can be so devastating in poor countries is that malnutrition leaves the stomach lining inflamed (gastritis) and acid secretion dangerously impaired. But even in the midst of plenty, we may be leaving ourselves vulnerable to serious bacterial GI infections simply by following "doctor's orders," that is, by taking antacids and acid suppressors.

As far back as 1885, the pioneering German bacteriologist Robert Koch found he could promote cholera infections in guinea pigs simply by feeding them a dose of bicarbonate (which neutralizes normal stomach acid) prior to infecting them with the *V. cholerae*.[9] This works in people as well. Almost one-hundred years later, a study showed that healthy human volunteer "guinea pigs" could also increase their risk of cholera infection by first taking a dose of sodium bicarbonate.[10] (Even though cholera gets the most research attention as one of the most serious infectious gastrointestinal diseases, please remember that this discussion applies to *every* potential gastrointestinal infection, including the "mutant" *E. coli* OH157, the deadly meat-contaminant organism that appears to be a result of routinely feeding antibiotics to animals.)

One way that doctors may literally be killing people is by promoting bacterial infections with acid-suppressing drugs. It has become common practice in hospitals today to freely dispense drugs like Prilosec and Zantac to very sick patients, such as those in intensive care. The aim is to make them more comfortable (if they have heartburn or esophageal reflux) and to prevent "stress ulcers" from forming in the stomach.*

No doubt, the doctors who prescribe these drugs have the best of intentions, but the evidence suggests that their "approved" treatment pro

---

*By contrast, vitamin A helps *prevent* pneumonia and other infections.

motes pneumonia* development in a significant number of their patients. "Nosocomial" (hospital-caused) pneumonia—a bacterial infection of the lungs—is a huge problem in hospitals today, accounting for 17 percent of hospital-acquired infections. It increases length of stay in the hospital, helps send health care costs through the roof, and kills 50 percent of people who develop the disease while on a mechanical ventilator.[11]

In the vast majority of cases of hospital-acquired pneumonia, the bacteria that infect the lungs originate deep down in the GI tract. With normal acid levels in the stomach, there is little risk of bacteria from the intestines working their way up into the lungs. However, reduced stomach acid that may accompany critical illness, combined with drug-induced acid suppression and/or neutralization, can raise gastric pH to levels that encourage bacterial overgrowth and migration.

How do the bacteria get from the gut to the lungs? Small amounts of bacteria-laden gastric contents may get aspirated (inhaled) during episodes of reflux. Also, in seriously ill people, tubes placed into the airways, nose, mouth, and stomach can all serve as superhighways for disease-causing organisms.

Lots of research demonstrates that the risk of nosocomial pneumonia in critically ill people is significantly lower when they are treated, not with an acid suppressor, but with a mucosal protective agent (sucralfate) that coats the mucosal lining but does not alter gastric pH. In a study published in the *New England Journal of Medicine*, patients on mechanical ventilation were randomly divided into two groups. One group took either an H_2-receptor-blocking drug, a neutralizing antacid, or both, while the other group took just sucralfate. The rate of pneumonia was twice as high in the acid suppressor/neutralizer group as in the sucralfate group. The acid-suppressed people were also 60 percent more likely to die from pneumonia.[12]

"Stealing" Nutrients

In the previous chapter, we described how low acid directly inhibits the absorption of many vitamins, minerals, proteins, and amino acids. Bacterial overgrowth due to low stomach acid can also rob us of vital nutrients in a variety of other ways:[13]

---

*One research team has demonstrated that intravenously administered vitamin A reduced the occurrence of "stress ulceration" in severely stressed, hospitalized individuals from 63 percent to 18 percent (MS Chernov et al., "Stress Ulcer: A Preventable Disease." *J Trauma* 1972; 12:831–846). As vitamin A is not patentable, its use for this and other purposes has been less than emphasized by patent medicine companies.

- **Stealing vitamin B_{12}.** Some bacteria capture free vitamin B_{12} or vitamin B_{12}-protein complexes. Others produce "false vitamin B_{12}" (technically termed "vitamin B_{12} analog"), which competes with its regular counterpart for absorption, effectively diluting the actual vitamin B_{12}. These analogs can also interfere with certain forms of vitamin B_{12} testing, creating a false impression of "normal" levels.

- **Blocking fat absorption.** Fat malabsorption can occur when certain bacteria in the stomach break down bile salts (deconjugation) before they have a chance to metabolize the fat.

- **Carbohydrate malabsorption.** A number of mechanisms have been proposed to explain how bacteria in the stomach interfere with the absorption of sugars and other carbohydrates.

- **Water and nutrient loss.** Bacterial overgrowth in the upper GI tract can promote excessive loss of water and nutrients by causing chronic diarrhea.

How to Fill Your Stomach with Germs

Acid-suppressing drugs promote bacterial overgrowth, a fact that has been documented in numerous studies of people being treated for either GERD or duodenal ulcer.[14-25]

In one recent trial, thirty people with GERD were treated with high doses of Prilosec (40 mg/day) for at least three months. A control group included ten GERD patients not taking any acid suppressors at the time. When the researchers took samples of stomach juice from all the subjects, they found that eleven of the thirty Prilosec-treated people had developed bacterial overgrowth, compared with one of the ten people in the control group (see Figure 5-1). Bacterial overgrowth in the Prilosec group also interfered with bile acid metabolism.[26] Bile acids, which are produced in the liver and stored in the gall bladder, are required for normal fat digestion.

As we noted earlier, it has been known for more than a century that high intragastric pH permits bacteria to grow in the normally sterile stomach. Long-term use of Prilosec, one of the most potent acid-suppressing agents ever developed, reduces the secretion of HCl to near zero, resulting in a state of near-achlorhydria and a kind of "functional atrophic gastritis." Here is what the official, FDA- "approved" Prilosec Product Information states about the risk of bacterial overgrowth:

As do other agents that elevate intragastric pH, omeprazole [Prilosec] administered for 14 days in healthy subjects produced a significant increase in the intragastric concentrations of viable bacteria. The pattern of the bacterial species was unchanged from that commonly found in saliva. All changes resolved within three days of stopping treatment.[27]

What's curious about this statement is the way it downplays the significance of what is clearly an important side effect. The statement begins by pointing out that Prilosec is not the only guilty party here, since " . . . other agents that elevate gastric pH" also cause bacterial overgrowth. The implication seems to be that this makes it all right. Of course, this is nonsense. If bacterial overgrowth is an undesirable and potentially dangerous condition, then that's what it is. To suggest that it's not such a bad thing if lots of different drugs also cause it is self-serving and misleading.

The statement reflects the results of a rather limited (fourteen-day) clinical trial in "healthy subjects," that is, people without heartburn or other serious disease. Unfortunately, most people with indigestion, heartburn, or GERD take Prilosec for a lot longer than fourteen days. They may take it daily for months or years or even decades, because if they stop taking it, their indigestion and heartburn will almost certainly return. (Lest we forget, Prilosec does not *cure* anything; it just temporarily *suppresses* symptoms.) Moreover, people who take Prilosec in "real life" are probably not going to be as healthy as the paid volunteers in this controlled clinical trial. They will likely have long-standing indigestion and/or reflux causing heartburn and may have atrophic gastritis or other serious GI disorders. They may also be taking other drugs, their diet may be deficient in some important nutrients, and they may be less able to tolerate any added acid suppression.

The Prilosec statement also points out that most of the bugs found growing in the stomach come from the mouth (saliva), as if to say,

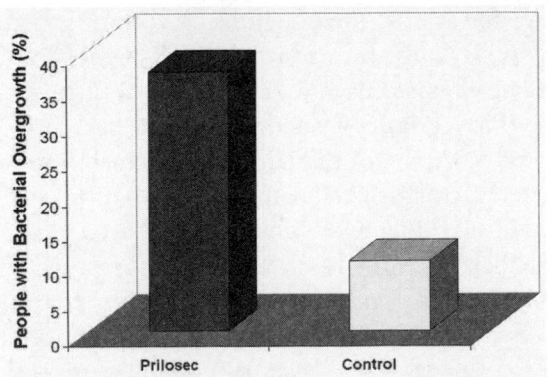

Figure 5-1. GERD patients treated with Prilosec (40 mg/day) for over 3 months showed significantly more bacterial overgrowth than a control group of GERD patients who were not taking acid-suppressing drugs. Adapted from Theisen et al., 2000.

"How bad could they be?" In fact (just ask your dentist), the normal, healthy mouth contains more than four-hundred different species of bacteria, amounting to billions and billions of microorganisms. As one dental researcher observed, "In one mouth, the number of bacteria can easily exceed the numbers of people who live on Earth."[28] More importantly, as we have discussed, some types of bacteria that enter the stomach via the nose or mouth could cause serious, even fatal, illness. Whether bacteria are benign or dangerous depends not just on the nature of the bugs themselves, but also on where they are located. Bacteria from the mouth (and the intestines) are supposed to be killed by acid when they enter the stomach. Allowing them to live in the stomach creates an unnatural condition with proven consequences for our health. The skin of most people is literally covered with bacteria called *Staphylococcus aureus*. We get along quite well with *Staph. aureus* as long as it stays *on* the skin. But should it get *under* the skin, or, worse, into the bloodstream, *Staph. aureus* can be deadly.

The Prilosec statement concludes by pointing out that bacterial growth ceases within 3 days after stopping the drug. That is certainly good news. The problem, of course, is that the way acid suppressors are promoted, prescribed, and used today, people don't stop taking them after three days. They often take them daily for months or years at a time, creating a chronic state of hypochlorhydria or achlorhydria.

Helicobacter pylori:
The Bug That Beats the Acid Test

While most bacteria are doomed to extinction once they encounter the acidic environment of a normal stomach, there is one, called *Helicobacter pylori*, that has found a way to live a long and happy life in the land of the low pH. Unfortunately, once established in the stomach, *H. pylori* becomes a serious threat to our health and longevity for a number of reasons:

- *H. pylori* is presently thought to be the leading cause of atrophic gastritis, accounting for 80 percent to 100 percent of cases.[29]

- *H. pylori* also causes the vast majority of gastric* (80 percent) and duodenal (95 percent) ulcers.[30]

---

*Gastric ulcers occur in the stomach, while duodenal uclers occur in the duodenum. Both types of ulcer are known collectively as peptic ulcers.

- *H. pylori* has been linked to two forms of stomach cancer: adenocarcinoma and lymphoma. According to results of large epidemiologic studies from both Europe and the United States, *H. pylori* infection increases the risk of gastric carcinoma by 600 percent and is responsible for 50 percent of all cases of adenocarcinoma.[31-32]

H. pylori protects itself from HCl in the stomach by a mechanism that mimics the way the stomach lining protects itself. The bacteria secrete an enzyme that results in the formation of ammonia and carbon dioxide, which in turn combine with water to produce ammonium *bicarbonate*. Bicarbonate molecules, of course, make excellent acid neutralizers. This means that *H. pylori*, bathing safely in its self-made neutralizing shield, is free to thrive and burrow its corkscrewlike body through the mucosal layer and into the gastric epithelium, where it is protected not just from stomach acid but from antibiotic drugs as well.

Exactly how *H. pylori* damages the stomach lining is still under investigation. Its damage can be diffuse (gastritis) or localized (ulcers). Depending on the location of the gastritis it causes, *H. pylori* infection can result in true hyperacidity (hyperchlorhydria) or a loss of stomach acid (hypochlorhydria or achlorhydria). When *H. pylori* infection is confined to the antrum of the stomach, the region where most of the gastrin-producing cells are located, it stimulates these G cells to work overtime making

Do You Have "Bowel Breath"?

From time to time, I'm consulted at Tahoma Clinic by individuals who mention (usually reluctantly) that one of their symptoms is "very bad breath," "incredibly bad breath," or in one memorable instance, "bowel breath," that won't go away with brushing, flossing, or mouthwash. By now, chances are good that you've guessed where "bowel breath" comes from. That's right: all those germs, uninhibited by stomach acid, making their happy home in the stomach and letting the world know by their odor!

and secreting gastrin. The excess gastrin circulates in the blood, and when it reaches the parietal cells, located farther north in the body and fundus, it prods them to turn on the acid spigots full blast. All this extra acid, helped along by an *H. pylori*-mediated reduction in bicarbonate production in the duodenum, is the primary irritant (but *not the cause*) in duodenal ulcers. The acid degrades the gastric mucosal layer laid bare by *H. pylori*. The resulting long-term irritation can lead to localized open sores called duodenal ulcers. Duodenal ulcers are one of the few GI disorders actually associated with excess stomach acid, or hyperacidity. (Notice we say "associated with" and not "caused by." That's because the *cause* of both the ulceration and the excess acidity is *H. pylori* itself.)

Most of the time, *H. pylori* sets up shop in the centrally located body (corpus) of the stomach. When this happens, a whole different pattern of pathology emerges. The resulting inflammation—atrophic gastritis—inhibits normal acid secretion from the parietal cells located there. Localized irritation may develop into peptic ulcers, even as acid levels fall. Once an area is damaged by *H. pylori*, it doesn't take much acid to make things worse. Prolonged atrophic gastritis and hypochlorhydria or achlorhydria can eventually develop into gastric cancer (see below). Thus, while acid suppression has long been a major treatment—sometimes the *only* treatment—for both duodenal and gastric ulcers, high acid levels are seen only with duodenal ulcers. Gastric ulcers occur *despite* low acid secretion. If this treatment doesn't work very well, it's not hard to see why.

Ulcers and Acid Suppression

This picture of peptic ulcers is actually a relatively recent discovery. Until the 1980s, conventional medicine considered ulcers to be a result of stress or other factors, which allowed "excess" stomach acid to *cause* the lesion. Although *H. pylori* was known to inhabit the stomach (called *Campylobacter pylori* at that time), few suspected that it had anything to do with ulcers.

In its time-(dis)honored fashion, though, the patent medicine industry took off after stomach acid as the "cause" of GI ulcers. Acid-suppressing drugs—from Tagamet to Prilosec—were initially developed to treat ulcers. Although they could often relieve some of the ulcer pain and discomfort and perhaps help slow their progression, the drugs could never "cure" ulcers, for the obvious reason that acid doesn't *cause* them. People with ulcers who took these drugs needed to take them forever, because as soon as they stopped taking them, their ulcers would almost certainly flare up again. (Also in the 1980s, research in England demonstrated that an inexpensive licorice compound actually healed ulcers as well as Tagamet, and prevented ulcer recurrence even better . . . but it wasn't patentable, so only people who visited natural food stores were ever informed about it. See chapter 7 for more about the healing power of licorice.)

The real breakthrough against ulcers came in the early 1980s when an Australian medical researcher, Barry Marshall, M.D., began presenting evidence that the actual cause of ulcers was *H. pylori*. With billions invested in acid-suppressing drugs, conventional medicine wanted nothing to do with Marshall's discoveries, and for the better part of a decade, they ignored and ridiculed them. (Where have we heard that refrain before?) Eventually, though, the weight of the evidence became too much to ignore, and *H. pylori* infection was finally acknowledged as the primary cause of peptic ulcers.

Why *H. pylori* and Prilosec Don't Mix

During the early 1990s, the focus of ulcer treatment began to shift away from acid suppression and toward *H. pylori* eradication, usually with antibiotic drugs. (There's an effective, inexpensive, and much safer natural treatment for *H. pylori*, too. More about this in chapter 7.) Nevertheless, acid suppression, usually with Prilosec, is still widely prescribed as an adjunct to antibiotics, the presumption being that reduced acid secretion permits more rapid healing.

Prilosec also remains the most widely prescribed drug for treating heartburn, indigestion, and related disorders. This, of course, is a vastly larger "market" for the drug than peptic ulcers ever were. The fact remains, though, that many people with symptoms of "acid indigestion" have *H. pylori* infections even though they do not have ulcers. Unfortunately, the practice of giving acid suppressors to people with *H. pylori* infection not only provides no therapeutic benefit (Prilosec does not kill or inhibit the bacteria), but it can actually make things much, much worse.

The reality is that reducing stomach acid makes life significantly easier for *H. pylori* and, therefore, significantly more dangerous for us. Several studies have shown that gastritis (inflammation) and epithelial lesions in the body (corpus) of the stomach *increases* when people infected with *H. pylori* take Prilosec or other acid-suppressing drugs.[33–39]

The dangers of mixing Prilosec and *H. pylori* were brought clearly home in a 1996 article published in the *New England Journal of Medicine*. The researchers, from Sweden and the Netherlands, followed (for a mean of five years) two groups of people who were being treated for reflux esophagitis. One group took Prilosec (20–40 mg/day) and the other underwent a surgical procedure called fundoplication, which repairs the

LES but does not involve acid suppression. Among those people who had documented *H. pylori* infections at the start of the study and who were treated with Prilosec, the rate of atrophic gastritis increased from 59 percent at the beginning of treatment to 81 percent by the end of the study (see Figure 5-2).[40] It is worth noting that, among those who had no atrophic gastritis at the start of the study, 30 percent of those who took Prilosec later developed it. By contrast, just 4 percent of the surgically treated group developed atrophic gastritis.

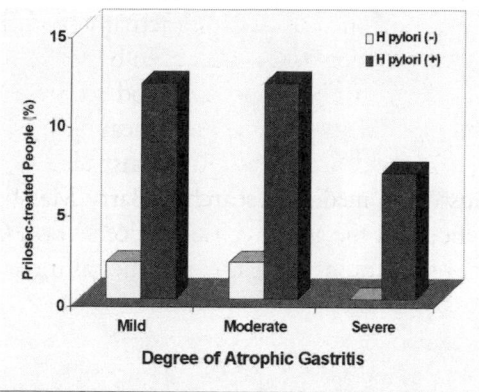

Figure 5-2. Development of atrophic gastritis in people, with or without *H. pylori* infection, who were treated for reflux esophagitis with Prilosec and who had no atrophic gastritis at baseline. Adapted from EJ Kuipers et al., 1996.

Advancing the Cancer Clock

Let's think about all this for a moment. Atrophic gastritis is a major risk factor for stomach cancer (as well as a host of other diseases related to acid suppression). *H. pylori* is the leading cause of atrophic gastritis. Taking an acid-suppressor on top of an *H. pylori* infection makes the bacteria an even greater threat to cause atrophic gastritis. Would it be too much to suggest, then, that taking an acid suppressor with *H. pylori* in the gut increases our risk of stomach cancer? We think not. Given this knowledge, it would be safe to say that these drugs should be classed as carcinogen-facilitators under these conditions. Prescribing these drugs without, at the very least, testing patients for *H. pylori* would appear to border on medical malpractice. How many doctors are testing their patients for *H. pylori* before reaching for their prescription pad at the first sign of heartburn? Precious few, we can be sure.

Although the Dutch/Swedish study appeared in one of the leading medical journals in the world, it seems to have caused barely a ripple. In an editorial accompanying the article, Julie Parsonnet, M.D., of Stanford University Medical School, writes: "In principle, current [acid-suppressing drug] therapies might be *advancing the cancer clock* by converting relatively benign gastric inflammation into a more destructive, premalignant process." She adds that while there was no convincing evidence that drug-induced acid suppression increases the risk of gastric cancer, "the long-term

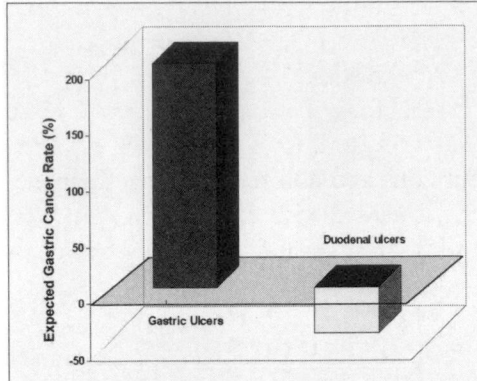

Figure 5-3. The ulcer-cancer paradox. Having duodenal ulcers (and excess gastric HCl) appears to preclude gastric cancer, while having gastric ulcers (and an HCl deficiency) increases the risk. Adapted from L-E Hansson et al., 1996.

use of acid-inhibiting therapy in patients with *H. pylori* infection should be *viewed with some caution*"[41] (emphasis added). Note that Dr. Parsonnet wrote these words in 1996, just a year before the widespread promotion of Prilosec for treating common heartburn began. Despite these cautions, the official Prescribing Information for Prilosec and other acid suppressors offers not even a hint that physicians or their patients might want to think about *H. pylori* before using these drugs.

Even more frightening is the fact that millions of people are now taking acid suppression into their own hands by using over-the-counter versions of Zantac, Pepcid, Axid, and Tagamet without even going to the doctor. Thus, they virtually eliminate any chance of discovering an *H. pylori* infection. We shudder to think ahead when decades of acid suppression begin to bear fruit in the form of an epidemic of stomach cancer.

How Acid Suppression Raises the Cancer Risk

There is a paradox that baffled medicine early in the nineteenth century. That is when it was first noticed that people who have *gastric* ulcers tend to get stomach cancer, while those with *duodenal* ulcers do not. Once the role of *H. pylori* infection in duodenal and gastric ulcers and atrophic gastritis was discovered in the 1980s and 1990s, the paradox took on another dimension: *H. pylori* could be the causative agent in either duodenal ulcers or gastric cancer, but hardly ever both at the same time. On the other hand, gastric ulcers and gastric cancer can occur simultaneously. The most recent confirmation of this paradox was a well-controlled U.S.-Swedish study that found twice the expected rate of gastric cancer in people who had gastric ulcers but 40 percent less than expected in those with duodenal ulcers (see Figure 5-3).[42]

How can this be? The likely answer lies in—you guessed it—gastric pH. Remember we mentioned earlier that duodenal ulcers were associated with *hyper*acidity, while gastric ulcers occur in an environment of hypochlorhydria or achlorhydria. A low gastric pH (remember low pH = high acidity) is the normal state of affairs for the stomach and could not be carcinogenic, even if acid levels were excessive. (If that *were* the case, the human species would have died out eons ago. On the other hand, an elevated pH—an unnatural condition associated with disease (e.g., *H. pylori* infection, atrophic gastritis)—is an important risk factor for gastric carcinoma.

There appear to be at least two major mechanisms by which hypochlorhydria and achlorhydria elevate the risk of stomach cancer: by raising gastrin levels (hypergastrinemia), and by promoting bacterial overgrowth.

Hypergastrinemia Speeds Up Mucosal Cell Growth

Hypergastrinemia (high gastrin levels in the blood) typically occurs in people with atrophic gastritis or in those who take acid-blocking drugs for long periods of time. The amount of gastrin in play at any one time is a direct reflection of the current level of stomach acid. Low acid levels (pH 3 or higher) in gastric atrophy trigger higher gastrin levels as the stomach tries to compensate for the loss of acidity. A standard 20-mg daily dose of Prilosec causes up to a three- to four-fold increase in gastrin levels.[43] In people whose heartburn/GERD fails to respond to the standard dose, long-term treatment with doses as high as 40 or 60 mg has produced gastrin levels as much as tenfold above normal.[44][47]

Chronically elevated gastrin is a concern due primarily to its ability to raise the risk of developing stomach cancer. The hormone normally promotes the growth and proliferation of new histamine-secreting ECL cells as well as acid-producing parietal cells in the lining of the stomach. A steady supply of new ECL and parietal cells is required to replace those that succumb to the hostile gastric environment, especially in the fundus, where acid levels are highest. Thus, turning up the gastrin flow not only increases stomach acid, but it also speeds up the ECL cell assembly lines. As long as the increase in gastrin matches the decrease in acid, everything hums along normally. But when the gastrin supply badly exceeds the demand, ECL cell growth may be excessive. Known as *hyperplasia*, excess ECL cell growth is common in people with atrophic gastritis and has been observed in people taking Prilosec as well.[48-49]

In some people, such growth can turn cancerous. This may be similar to the situation in women, where too much estrogen in the breast or uterus stimulates hyperplasia, which occasionally develops into cancer. There is currently no clear evidence that taking acid-suppressors for a long time directly causes stomach cancer. However, it is known that the risk increases in people with atrophic gastritis, which can take decades to develop fully. Few people have been using Prilosec or other even more powerful PPIs regularly for more than six or seven years, so far.

If rat studies are a lesson, though, long-term use of acid-suppressing drugs may indeed be risky. In one study, twenty-four months of use caused a statistically significant dose-related increase in ECL hyperplasia and gastric carcinoid tumors (known as ECLomas).[50] When people take Prilosec for up to five years, examination has revealed a positive correlation between precancerous changes in the stomach lining and the degree of atrophic gastritis.[51-52] No cases of stomach cancer have been attributed outright to the use of Prilosec or any other acid suppressor yet, however.

Carcinoid tumors are usually less serious than adenocarcinomas, but they can still be troublesome and extremely dangerous. This is because they flood the body with gastrin, which responds with a virtual flood of stomach acid. In the condition known as *Zollinger-Ellison Syndrome* (ZES), carcinoid-induced hypergastrinemia leads to extremely high gastric acid levels. All that acid eventually overpowers the stomach's natural acid protections and leads to the formation of multiple severe ulcers, especially in the duodenum.[53] ZES is one of the few conditions known in which stomach acid levels are actually too high.

Dramatic hypergastrinemia is also a key symptom of the disease known as *pernicious anemia*, which is associated with severe atrophic gastritis and malabsorption of vitamin B_{12}, as well as both carcinoid tumors and gastric adenocarcinomas. In pernicious anemia, atrophic gastritis is so severe that parietal cells lose the ability to secrete not only acid, but *intrinsic factor* also. Since both HCl and intrinsic factor are required for the digestion and absorption of vitamin B_{12}, malabsorption results.

Numerous reports have been published relating cases of hypergastrinemia in people with achlorhydria/pernicious anemia who were treated with high doses of Prilosec.[54-59] As one author reviewing the published scientific literature on elevated gastrin levels understated, "The evidence indicates that chronic hypergastrinemia may not be totally benign."[60]

Elevated gastrin may also be a factor in some cases of *human colorectal cancer*, although the data are much fuzzier than they are for gastric adenocarcinoma. Nevertheless, it appears that the risk of developing carcinoids and gastric adenocarcinoma due to chronic hypergastrinemia may be increased if one possesses a specific gene. Whether acid-suppressing drugs can contribute to colorectal cancer remains "up in the air" at this time.[61]

Stomach Acid and Cancer: The Bacterial Link

We have known about the link between low stomach acid levels and gastric cancer since as early as 1879. That was when physicians, mainly in Germany, first began reporting their observations that people with stomach cancer almost always had little or no HCl in their stomachs.[62] More systematic studies over the years have confirmed that atrophic gastritis, in association with achlorhydria or serious hypochlorhydria, is a major risk factor for stomach cancer. And the risk increases with the severity of the gastritis and the length of time a person has it.[63] In one Danish study, people with the most severe atrophic gastritis had a four- to sixfold increased risk of developing gastric cancer. In some cases, it took up to seventeen years after achlorhydria was diagnosed for cancer to develop. In three cases, it took more than nine years.[64]

How does atrophic gastritis develop into cancer? No one knows for sure, but the missing link may be bacterial overgrowth. According to the most widely accepted theory, some bacteria (but not *H. pylori*) are able to turn *nitrate* molecules, found commonly in food, into *nitrite* molecules. Noted one review of the scientific research on this connection, "This is a powerful hypothesis which is supported by much experimental evidence."[65]

Nitrites were once widely used to cure, or preserve, meats such as bacon and ham. But in the 1970s, it was discovered that a *healthy* stomach can convert nitrites to chemicals called *nitrosamines*, which are known to be carcinogenic. As a result, nitrites are used far less often in food preservation today.

Nevertheless, nitrites produced in the stomach by bacteria from nitrates in ordinary food can be just as dangerous as the ones we get from a charbroiled bacon burger. Studies have shown that the concentration of nitrite in gastric juice rises along with the pH and the extent of bacterial overgrowth. People with chronic atrophic gastritis and hypochlorhydria make significantly more nitrite from dietary nitrate compared with healthy controls.[66]

Given these reactions, it should come as no surprise that taking acid-suppressing drugs raises nitrite and nitrosamine concentrations. In people taking Tagamet for peptic ulcers, for example, a 73 percent reduction in basal acid secretion resulted in statistically significant increases in nitrites and nitrosamines. Even when the dose was reduced to a maintenance level for three months, nitrite and nitrosamine concentrations remained elevated, suggesting the presence of a prolonged carcinogenic stimulus.[67]

Direct evidence that the prolonged use of acid-suppressing drugs increases the risk of gastric cancer has been limited and difficult to interpret. Use of some acid-suppressing drugs but not others has been reported to cause gastric malignancy in laboratory animals, but extrapolation from rats to humans is always fraught with difficulties.[68]

Anecdotal reports of gastric carcinomas in people taking Tagamet for ulcers began appearing shortly after the drug was introduced.[69-71] In a very large study comparing nearly ten thousand Tagamet users with more than nine thousand controls, the death rate and the incidence of GI cancers were both significantly higher in the Tagamet-treated group, although it appeared at the time that most of the malignancies could be explained more easily by other causes.[72] In another survey of about seventeen thousand Tagamet users, the risk of cancer was found to be ten times greater than expected. However, these results were also difficult to interpret, because the risk declined overall with further use, while it increased in women taking the drug for seven years or longer.[73-74]

If A = B and B = C, Does A = C?

Absent any direct proof that acid-suppressing drugs may lead to gastric cancer, we need to fall back on the circumstantial findings. For example, there is no doubt that acid suppression promotes bacterial overgrowth and that bacterial overgrowth promotes production of carcinogenic nitrosamine compounds. There is also no doubt that acid-suppressing drugs increase the progression and severity of atrophic gastritis in people with *H. pylori* infection, and that atrophic gastritis is a major risk factor for gastric carcinoma. Commenting on these risks in 1989, before Prilosec use had become as widespread as it is now, one researcher wrote: "Until information is available about the effects of powerful gastric secretory inhibitors on the proliferative indices and patterns of the human mucosa, the drugs *must be categorized as too dangerous to use therapeutically*, especially since the proposed therapeutic benefits are minimal"[75] (emphasis added).

A Prediction

We want to be clear: At this time, there is *no outright proof* that prolonged use of acid-suppressing drugs causes cancer. Given all the presently known facts, however, we find it quite reasonable to predict that (if the possibility is seriously studied) at least some acid-suppressing drugs will be found to significantly increase the risk of cancer, especially if they are used for a long time.

CHAPTER 6
How Low Stomach Acid Can Make You Sick:
Asthma, Rheumatoid Arthritis, and Other Diseases

"It appears to me not unreasonable that the poison, as it may be called, which is generated by food ill assimilated, finds its way into the circulation; and hence arises the misery of hereditary asthma."
> —H. L. Pridham, "Observations on
> the Treatment of Asthma,"
> Br Med J. *1860;1:434–435*

"We're here to finish off Bobby's asthma," Rebecca Cutler declared. "He's lots better already, but we can't do it all ourselves. We've done everything you told the Pizzolis to do for their son, Vincent, and it's working! We're all members of the same church, Bobby and Vincent are classmates, and when Vincent's asthma disappeared in three months, we couldn't believe it. So we decided to try."

"And Bobby's asthma is more than halfway gone," his father, David, added. "I think we just need that injectable vitamin B_{12}, some allergy work, that test for his stomach, and maybe we can get it gone completely. At least we hope so. Bobby's had a tough time . . . we've had to rush him to the emergency room five times in just the last two years. Since we started as much of Vincent's program as we could, he's off the theophylline. That stuff made him 'hyper' all the time and made his heart race. He still needs to use his inhaler fairly often, but his wheezing is a lot less when it happens, and it goes away easier. And he's sleeping better at night, not waking up near as much."

I turned to Bobby. "What have Mom and Dad had you doing about your asthma lately, Bobby?"

"I can't have any more milk or cheese or ice cream, and I hafta take a bunch of vitamins and stuff." He looked worried. "Do I hafta take shots every day like Vincent?"

"Is your asthma better since you stopped drinking milk and started taking your vitamins like Vincent?"

"Yeah."

"Then it's possible that shots might help you like Vincent, too, isn't it?" Bobby looked dubious. "I guess."

"I can't tell you for sure they'll work, Bobby, but it sounds likely." I turned back to his parents. His mother handed me a list.

"Here's a summary of what we're doing so far," she said. "Bobby's seven, the same as Vincent, so we just gave him the same, as much as we could."

I read from the list. "Let's see: no milk or dairy products of any kind. All other foods, each one eaten only every four days or less . . . "

"We did it that way 'cause we have no idea exactly what foods Bobby's allergic to yet," Rebecca said. "But Monica, Vincent's mother, told me you said no cow's milk or dairy under any circumstances. And you asked her to 'rotate' Vincent's less-allergic foods every four days. So we made everything every four days until we had him tested."

"Makes sense." I resumed reading the list. "Vitamin B_{12}, 1000 micrograms three times a day, magnesium, 125 milligrams three times daily; vitamin B_6, 50 milligrams three times daily. . . . "

"The Pizzolis said vitamin B_{12} should be injected, but since it's harmless, we thought we'd try having Bobby swallow it anyway until we could see you. They also said that building up tissue magnesium levels reduces the tendency to muscle spasm, including bronchial muscle," David remarked.

"Exactly. Let's see: vitamin C, 1000 milligrams three times daily; one tablespoon of cod liver oil daily, and a high-potency multiple vitamin-mineral, one-third the adult quantity, three times daily. Everything in capsules, not tablets."

"That's because most asthmatic children have poor digestion, and capsules usually digest better than some tablets, right?" Rebecca asked.

"Right on both, though it's not 100 percent on either."

"Also, we threw every bit of sugar, refined carbohydrate, hydrogenated vegetable oil, and food chemicals out of the house," Rebecca said. "Monica told me you recommend doing that no matter what the problem is, and also just for staying as healthy as possible."

"Absolutely!" I replied. "None of those items have any place in healthful diets."

"Takes some getting used to, but since we did, I've felt less tired," David observed.

"Let's check Bobby over, and then have lab tests done, with your permission, of course," I said.

"That's what we brought Bobby here for," David said. "Monica said that food allergies are more important than inhalant allergies in childhood asthma, and you'd check both. But I didn't understand what testing his stomach has to do with asthma. Could you explain?"

"Sure. In a 1931 publication, Dr. George Bray, an asthma specialist, noted that 80 percent of two hundred asthmatic children had underproduction of acid and pepsin in the stomach. This, of course, impairs digestion, lowering nutrient absorption, and gradually increasing allergies to foods. In 1979, other researchers published proof that food allergy, particularly cow's milk, can cause the stomach problem in the first place."

"So it's sort of circular . . . food allergy causes the stomach to malfunction, which leads to more food allergy and asthma."

"For approximately 80 percent of asthmatic children."

"And injecting vitamin B_{12} instead of just swallowing it?"

"Stomach malfunction impairs vitamin B_{12} nutrition. Also, in the late 1940s and early 1950s, extra vitamin B_{12} by injection was found to be very helpful in most cases of childhood asthma."

"How often does all of this work?"

"I can only give you approximations, but about 50 percent completely eliminate their wheezing, about 30 percent have major improvement, about 10 percent only minor improvement, and only about 10 percent no change."

"And I've read the death rate from asthma has been climbing the last few years," Rebecca remarked.

Six months later, Bobby's wheezing was gone. Although I recommended lifetime exclusion of cow's milk and dairy products, the large majority of his food and inhalant allergies had been desensitized, and his mother had liberalized his diet, while keeping all the "junk" out. His was taking capsules of hydrochloric acid and pepsin to aid his digestion, and vitamin B_{12} injections were down to a maintenance level. He continued his other oral supplements. Several years later, he remains free of asthmatic wheezing.*

· · ·

In the previous chapter, we discussed a variety of illnesses that can result from chronically low stomach acid secretion. Most of these, like gastric cancer and bacterial infections, are diseases of the GI system itself. But the consequences of low stomach acid can extend far beyond the GI tract. In this chapter, we describe how a large number of serious diseases that appear—on the surface, at least—to be totally divorced from the workings of the stomach and intestines, may sometimes have their roots in a shortage of stomach acid. And, yes, restoring normal GI function can often yield remarkable degrees of improvement.

As we can see in the box on page 103, these are all dangerous and debilitating diseases, conditions that are notoriously difficult or impossible to treat effectively by conventional means. Most practitioners using conventional patent medicines would never connect these with low stomach acid.

Conventional medicine is anchored to the belief that synthetic symptom-suppressing drugs are nearly always the best therapy for most diseases. Thus, the standard treatment for inflammatory diseases, including allergies, asthma, rheumatoid arthritis, ulcerative colitis, and many others, consists primarily of powerful "anti-inflammatory" drugs that bring about temporary relief by *suppressing* the inflammation. Whatever it is that's *causing* the inflammatory reaction in the first place is usually completely ignored.

Yet, if we look beneath the surface symptoms, we find a common thread, a thread based in a majority of cases on fundamental molecular and genetic research. Investigators of human DNA have identified a complex of genes termed "histocompatibility locus antigens" (HLA) that

---

*Reprinted from Dr. Jonathan V. Wright's *Nutrition & Healing* newsletter, Agora South LLC, Baltimore, Maryland 21201, (410) 223-2611.

Diseases That May Be Related to Deficient Stomach Acid

Acne rosacea	Multiple sclerosis
Addison's disease	**Myasthenia gravis**
Allergic reactions	Osteoporosis
Celiac disease	**Pernicious anemia**
Childhood asthma	**Polymyalgia rheumatica**
Chronic autoimmune hepatitis	Reynaud's syndrome
Diabetes (type I–Juvenile)	Rheumatoid arthritis
Eczema (severe)	**Scleroderma**
Gallbladder disease	**Sjögren's syndrome**
Graves' disease (hyperthyroid)	**Ulcerative colitis**
Lupus erythematosus	**Vitiligo**
Macular degeneration	

appear to regulate many features of immunity. Furthermore, they have found that many diseases appear to "cluster" more frequently according to "HLA type."

All of the diseases listed in the box in **bold type** have been found by various investigators to cluster more frequently in the HLA types DR3, DR4, and B8. This means that even though these diseases and their symptoms may appear very different on the surface, on the genetic and molecular level they share at least one (and probably many more) common features. A major "common thread" in all these diseases is a dysfunction of the upper GI tract. Although not found in 100 percent of cases of the diseases listed above, it is usually found (if looked for) in over 50 percent of those diagnosed with each disease.*

More importantly, we find that by simply (and safely) restoring normal gastric function, many people with these diseases experience "amazing" improvement. These treatments do not suppress any symptoms. Instead, they help *alleviate the cause* of the inflammation or other symptoms. This distinction is extremely important. As an analogy, imagine a splinter in your foot is causing you pain and discomfort. You could take a pain-killing drug (temporary symptom suppression) or you could take the splinter out (remove the cause of the problem). Which solution makes more sense?

---

*This molecular and genetic commonality goes well beyond affecting just the upper GI tract. For example, appropriate use of the androgens DHEA and testosterone is very often beneficial in all of the HLA-linked diseases.

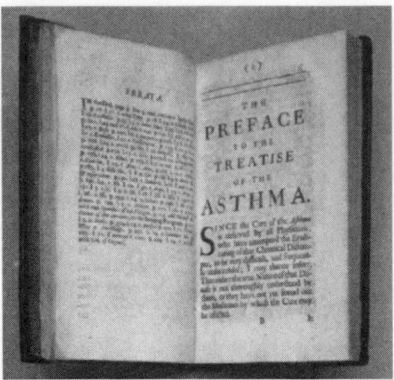

Figure 6-1. The 1698 *A Treatise of the Asthma* contains the first mention that impaired gastric function, later shown to be low stomach acid, might be a cause of asthma. *From the National Library of Medicine.*

Asthma

Asthma (especially childhood asthma) and stomach acid? People are often surprised to hear that this serious and increasingly common respiratory disorder, in which the airways become inflamed and constricted, making breathing difficult, may often begin in the stomach.

Most physicians routinely ignore the connection, remaining totally unaware of a medical literature linking asthma and stomach trouble that goes back more than *300 years*. In fact, the earliest mention of a gastric deficiency in asthma appeared in the very first medical text ever published in English on the subject of asthma. Sir John Floyer's *A Treatise of the Asthma* (see Figure 6-1), which first appeared in London in 1698, reported a "defect" in stomach juices. Wrote Floyer, "This defect of digestion and mucilaginous slime in the stomach are very obvious and observed by writers, and *were supposed the immediate cause of the asthma.*" (emphasis added).

Although we know today that asthma is a complex disease with multiple potential causes and triggers, there should be little doubt that low stomach acid can often play an important role. One of the most important scientific contributions in the modern age was a research report published in 1931 by the English physician Dr. George W. Bray, from the Asthma Clinic at the Hospital for Sick Children in London. In an era before the patent medicine industry became the driving force behind most medical research, Dr. Bray examined the stomach contents of more than two hundred children, aged six months to twelve years, who came to his hospital wheezing from asthma. He recovered gastric juice at regular intervals after a meal via a small tube passed into the children's stomachs. As his cases accumulated, he soon saw a pattern developing: (see Figure 6-2).[1]

- Overall, 80 percent of the asthmatic children had below normal acid secretion in their stomachs
- 23 percent had mild hypochlorhydria
- 48 percent had pronounced hypochlorhydria
- 9 percent had achlorhydria

As Dr. Bray followed these children for many years, he noticed that the acid deficiency was most pronounced in children under the age of seven years. As they grew older, though, many of the children's acid secretion returned to normal, which often coincided with the remission, or "spontaneous cure," of their asthma.

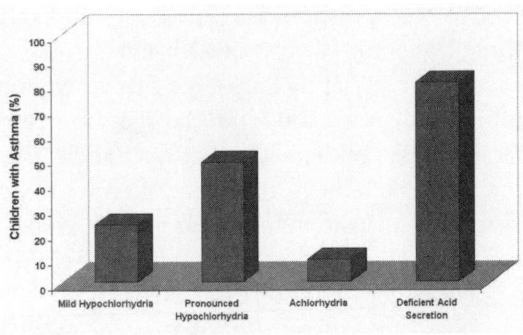

Figure 6-2. Repeated sampling of the stomach contents of more than two hundred children with asthma revealed varying degrees of acid deficiency in the vast majority of cases. Adapted from Bray, 1931.

Even today, physicians who treat children with asthma are well aware how common it is for them to "outgrow" their asthma as they pass through puberty and beyond. About half of all asthmatic children experience spontaneous remissions as they enter their teens.[2] One of the few investigations since Bray that has tried to understand why this happens reported that "spontaneous remission" occurred only in children when there was "no obvious cause" for their asthma. Could these children have had low stomach acid that returned to normal? We wouldn't be surprised, but we'll never know, because the researchers never looked.[3]

When George Bray found that so many of his asthma patients had low stomach acid, he did the logical thing: he had them replace the missing acid by taking a dilute solution of HCl and pepsin before or during their meals. What he found would be considered impossible by the standards of conventional asthma treatment. Over the course of three months, the acid therapy alone resulted in the children's eating better, gaining weight, and wheezing less. Eventually, their asthma attacks ceased altogether. "The child then appears perfectly well whilst taking the medicine," wrote Bray. But, he noted, if they stopped the acid therapy or caught a cold, they might suffer some mild attacks.

Even more impressive was what happened when Bray not only replaced the acid, but also limited the children's exposure to the allergens that were triggering their attacks. Their improvement was immediate. If the children continued to take their medicine throughout the winter, they remained asthma-free and could then safely discontinue the treatment.[4] This sounds suspiciously like a cure. If these children had been put on conventional anti-inflammatory corticosteroids and bronchodilators, they would not have been cured, but would likely have become dependent on these drugs for the rest of their lives.

It is an unhappy fact of life that conventional medicine, with its single-minded focus on drug-induced symptom suppression, doesn't know what to make of children who get over their asthma *without the help of drugs*. Such people may be regarded, often with a considerable degree of skepticism, as "curiosities." As their asthma wanes, they stop going to the doctor, who is usually too busy with "sick" children to follow up on those who somehow get better on their own.

Nor can we count on the patent medicine industry to find out why asthma goes away by itself so often. They've got too much invested in life-long symptom suppression to spend much of their considerable resources on investigating something that might lead to a real cure and would make their symptom suppressors obsolete. They're especially uninterested if the potential "cure" is a natural—and therefore *unpatentable*—substance like HCl, pepsin, or vitamin B_{12}, which would not earn them enormous profits. (Never lose sight of the fact that pharmaceutical companies are not in business to cure diseases, but rather to make money for their stockholders. Once a patient is cured, that patient doesn't need to buy any more drugs. But if his or her symptoms are suppressed, they may be "hooked" on the drugs for life.)

Most physicians never suspect that many of the children they see who "outgrew" their asthma might have done so because their gastric secretions gradually normalized with age. As a result, they don't have a clue that they might be able to hasten the disappearance of asthma by providing the children's stomachs what they're missing. They don't have a clue, because they don't know enough to look in the children's stomachs. Hardly any physicians measure intragastric pH on a routine basis, especially in cases of asthma. If they did, they'd be astounded! Children over age six (usually the youngest able to have their stomach acid accurately tested) with asthma have an approximate 50 percent to 60 percent incidence of mildly to severely low stomach acid. "Indirect" indicators of low stomach acid (the best easily available for very young children) suggest an even higher incidence of low stomach acid, approaching the 80 percent figure previously reported by Dr. George Bray.

Adults with asthma commonly have reflux esophagitis and GERD (see below). However, their diagnoses are often made by measuring *esophageal* pH, not *gastric* pH. Remember, excess acid in the esophagus *does not* necessarily signal excess acid in the stomach. In fact, all too often, excess esophageal acidity is associated with *too little* stomach acid.

Measuring stomach acidity is quite simple, and the information it provides is extremely valuable. The test we use to measure stomach acid secretion is described in chapter 7. It should be an essential part of any thorough medical examination. Unfortunately, it hardly ever is.

Permanent Natural Asthma Relief . . . Without Drugs

In my thirty years of clinical practice, I have found that about 50 percent of all children who come to the Tahoma Clinic with asthma find permanent relief of their wheezing within thirty to sixty days, without taking corticosteroid and bronchodilator drugs. Here's what we do:

- **Inject vitamin B_{12}, which is poorly absorbed when stomach acid, pepsin, and intrinsic factor are deficient (see chapter 4).** Frequently, the amounts of vitamin B_{12} needed to eliminate wheezing are (relatively) large, but, fortunately, vitamin B_{12} is quite safe.

- **Restore the stomach to normal function by replacing HCl and pepsin.** Although acid and pepsin are required to free up vitamin B_{12} from its protein carriers and thus allow for better absorption, it's likely that improving the digestion is just as important for reducing the occurrence of food allergies, which are the principal offenders in most case of childhood asthma.

- **Pay close attention to food allergies, especially to cow's milk.** Such allergies may result in varying degrees of allergic gastritis, leading to hypochlorhydria, low pepsin secretion, and possible failure to produce intrinsic factor.

- **Supplement magnesium and vitamin B_6,** both of which have been shown to lessen the severity and frequency of asthmatic attacks.

The Crucial Role of Vitamin B_{12} in Childhood (and Other) Forms of Asthma

The first hint that vitamin B_{12} might be useful against wheezing came serendipitously in 1949.[5] Again, it was a lone physician investigating the effect of vitamin B_{12} on "growth failure" in children in an Ohio camp. He

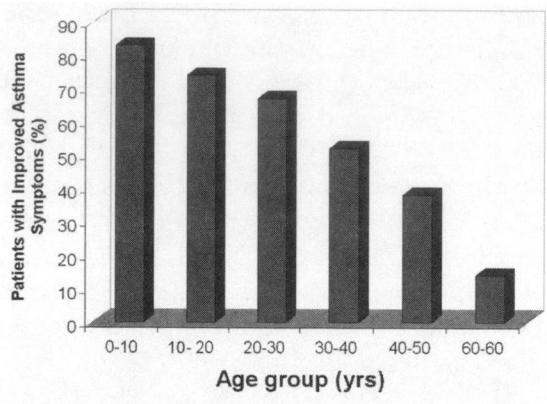

Figure 6-3. Effect of vitamin B_{12} on people with asthma. The percentage of people with asthma whose symptoms improved with vitamin B_{12} treatment is extremely high in youth but declines with advancing age. Adapted from Crockett, 1957.

gave the children capsules containing 10 micrograms of crystalline vitamin B_{12} each day to test whether it would promote growth. One of the children at the camp had what was described as "intractable" asthma with constant wheezing day and night. Within a week after the child started taking vitamin B_{12}, though, his asthmatic wheezing had vanished.

Two years later in another small trial, twenty adults with "intractable" asthma were given injections of 1000 micrograms of vitamin B_{12} once a week. After four weeks, eighteen of them reported improvement in breathing (although some wheezing remained), sleep, and in their general condition.[6]

An Italian study that was later abstracted in the *Journal of the American Medical Association* in 1952 reported the effects of daily intravenous injections of very high doses of vitamin B_{12} (30 *milli*grams, equal to 30,000 *micrograms*; fortunately it's nearly impossible to overdose with vitamin B_{12}) in twelve adults with asthma. After fifteen to twenty days, wheezing completely ceased in 83 percent (ten of twelve) of the study participants. Of the ten who were completely relieved, two later had a relapse, which responded to a repeat of the vitamin B_{12} treatment.[7]

In 1957, the English physician JA Crockett reported on a study he ran involving eighty-five people of all ages who had asthma.[8] All were given intramuscular injections of 1000 micrograms (1 milligram) of vitamin B_{12}, first at weekly intervals, and later at unspecified intervals up to four weeks. Using a four-level scoring system ("no change," "slight improvement," "moderate improvement," and "marked improvement") Dr. Crockett observed improvement in 56 percent (forty-eight out of eighty- five) of his test subjects. He also found that the ability to improve varied with age. It was extremely high in young children (83 percent) but declined with age. Even in the fifth and sixth decades of life, though, B_{12} injections resulted in nearly 40 percent improvement (see Figure 6-3).[9]

Based on these and other medical reports concerning vitamin B_{12} therapy, in 1976 we started advising parents to give their asthmatic children daily vitamin B_{12} injections, 500 to 3000 micrograms daily (depending on the child's age and weight). We have found that within thirty days of treatment, 50 percent stop wheezing entirely, and another 30 percent improve from a little to a lot. The injections are then tapered according to response, resuming or increasing again if the wheezing returns or becomes more severe again.

Parents understandably inquire about oral instead of injectable vitamin B_{12} treatment. If wheezing isn't severe, there's no reason not to try the "oral route" first. If it doesn't work (which is frequent) we can then proceed to injection.

Vitamin B_{12} *does not* work immediately to clear a particular wheezing episode. (A relatively rapid intravenous injection of magnesium accompanied by vitamin B_6 is much more effective in clearing acute wheezing.) Parents usually report improvement in chronic wheezing beginning after five to seven days of daily B_{12} shots. "Full results" and a "maintenance level" are usually reached after approximately thirty days.

Although vitamin B_{12} can eliminate or dramatically lessen the wheezing of childhood asthma, it *does not* eliminate the allergies that trigger attacks, nor does it repair the frequently underlying stomach problem, or restore the rest of the nutrients not getting absorbed due to poor gastric function. All these possible problems present in childhood asthma must be vigorously pursued or the afflicted child won't be as healthy as possible.

Asthma and Gastric Reflux: What's the Connection?

The success of HCl, pepsin, and vitamin B_{12} therapy suggests that the roots of asthma lie not in the lungs, where the symptoms appear, but in the stomach, where acid secretion and vitamin B_{12} digestion may be compromised. True to form, though, the patent medicine industry has largely ignored this lead and, instead, focused its considerable resources directly on symptom suppression in the lungs.

The result has been the development and widespread use of powerful—and dangerous—corticosteroids (e.g., prednisone, beclomethasone, triamcinolone), bronchodilators (e.g., albuterol, ephedrine, theophylline), and other drugs that are designed to suppress inflammation and dilate constricted airways. Thanks to thousands of pharmaceutical industry–sponsored research studies and hundreds of millions of dollars in advertising, promotion, and "education," about the only thing most physicians today know about asthma therapy is this kind of symptom suppression. They are taught to view asthma as a sometimes-"incurable" illness that can be "controlled" only by using anti-inflammatory and bronchodilator drugs (as well as inhalant allergy control). The cause(s) of asthma are not addressed by this approach. Although factors such as allergic reactions, airway "hyperreactivity," and a genetic predisposition are certainly important, the roles of low stomach acidity and deficient vitamin B_{12} are completely "off the radar screen" today.

Nevertheless, there is a growing awareness in conventional medicine that what goes on in the stomach does have something to do with the symptoms of asthma. In just the last ten years, more than four hundred scientific articles concerned with the connection between asthma and gastric acidity have been published. It turns out that one of the most common features of asthma, in addition to wheezing, is gastroesophageal reflux, often a sign of *low* stomach acid. It is estimated that between 30 percent and 89 percent of people with asthma also have GERD. Compared with healthy people, those with asthma also have significantly more reflux episodes and more acid-induced irritation of their esophageal lining.[10]

What is the connection between reflux and asthma? No one knows for sure, but it is certainly complex. It is unclear, for example, whether acid reflux causes asthma, whether asthma causes reflux, or whether both result from a common cause, such as low gastric acidity or activity in the vagus nerve, which serves both the gut and the airways.

It is known that drugs that are commonly used to treat asthma, such as the bronchodilators *theophylline*, *albuterol*, *ephedrine*, and *pseudoephedrine*, can weaken the LES valve, and thus promote acid reflux. It has also been suggested that the act of wheezing places added pressure on the LES during expiration, causing it to leak acidic gastric juice back into the esophagus.[11-13]

Do any of these mechanisms suggest that people with asthma have too much HCl in their stomachs? Of course not. As we have pointed out *ad nauseum* (no pun intended), excess acidity is relatively uncommon and is usually associated with conditions such as duodenal ulcer and Zollinger-Ellison syndrome. It is far more likely that people with asthma, especially children, have too little gastric acid. Unfortunately, although low stomach acid is often associated with reflux, *stomach* pH is virtually never measured in people with GERD let alone those with asthma. Most researchers are satisfied to report that *esophageal* acidity is elevated, but this hardly qualifies as news, nor is it particularly meaningful. Certainly, the pH in the esophagus will be more acidic than it should be. That is the definition of acid reflux. However, it tells us nothing about the amount of acid the stomach is secreting, just that the LES valve is malfunctioning.

Even so, to conventional medicine, the co-occurrence of reflux and asthma is becoming yet another reason to prescribe powerful acid suppressing drugs. Here's the rationale: It is not unusual for refluxed gastric juice to be inhaled (aspirated) into the lungs, especially when reflux occurs during sleep. In susceptible individuals, the acidic material might trigger an asthmatic reaction. Studies show that when acid gets into the windpipe, there is a tenfold drop in the ability of lungs to take in and breathe out air.[14-15] The operative theory is that, if acid reflux is triggering asthmatic attacks, then removing the acid should relieve the asthma.

Does this theory hold up? Not really. Several studies have investigated the use of Prilosec in people with asthma and GERD, and the results have been equivocal, at best. In general, improvement in pulmonary function, if and when it occurs, tends to be modest and is seen only at very high doses that virtually eliminate all stomach acid secretion. The standard therapeutic dose of Prilosec for GERD, 20 mg once a day, produces no improvement in asthma symptoms (e.g., wheezing and "airway constriction") or pulmonary lung function.[16] After six weeks of treatment, a dose of 40 mg, *twice* the daily dose, resulted in just a 20 percent improvement in the amount of forcefully exhaled air (a standard measure of pulmonary function) in 27 percent (fifteen out of fifty-six) of people with asthma and GERD.[17] In a third trial, a dose of 40 mg twice daily (*four* times the standard GERD dose) yielded only a small, but statistically significant, improvement in lung function after three months, but the patients continued to wheeze and to need bronchodilators and other medications as much as ever.[18] A European study using the same very high dose of Prilosec in thirty-six people with GERD and asthma found "no beneficial effect" on any measure of pulmonary function, despite producing what was described as a "profound effect on acid reflux." The researchers, from The Netherlands, concluded that their results " . . . *do not support a role for intensive anti-reflux therapy to improve pulmonary symptoms and function in patients with asthma . . . who have airway hyperresponsiveness despite maintenance treatment with inhaled corticosteroids*"[19] (emphasis added.)

A review of studies on acid-suppressing drugs published over thirty years (1966–1996) in major medical journals found that overall, asthma symptoms improved in 69 percent of people with GERD, asthma medication use dropped in 62 percent, and evening expiratory ability improved in 26 percent. *And yet, not one person showed significant improvement in lung function.* The authors concluded that acid-suppressing drug treatment "improves asthma symptoms, may reduce asthma medication use, *but has minimal or no effect on lung function*"[20] (emphasis added.)

Hardly a ringing endorsement! Yet, physicians who hear about patent medicine company–sponsored research by reading patent medicine–sponsored journals or Web sites, by going to patent medicine company–sponsored conventions, by taking *required* patent medicine company–sponsored Continuing Medical Education (CME) courses,* or by accepting "free" drug samples are beginning to get the message that some improvement might be possible in some patients whose asthma may be resistant to corticosteroid treatment. As a result, some physicians, such as allergists and family physicians, who may have no specific expertise in GI medicine, are beginning to prescribe Prilosec and other acid-suppressors "off-label" to their asthma patients. Sometimes they may prescribe the drug even if the patient doesn't complain of "acid indigestion," under the presumption that the reflux may be "silent" in some cases.[21-22]

It's a safe bet that these doctors give nary a thought to what the resulting acid suppression may be doing to their patients' stomachs, not to mention their general health. Do they actually measure stomach acid levels? Do they even measure esophageal pH? Do they ever test for atrophic gastritis, for *H. pylori* infection, or for vitamin/mineral malabsorption?

Of course not. In the vast majority of cases, the approach is empiric: Try the drug. If it works, fine, prescribe it forever. As one researcher has noted, "Because [GERD] is a chronic and unrelenting disease, aggressive therapy may be a lifetime commitment."[23] If all these drugs do is eliminate the stomach acid "nuisance," what could be the harm in that?

Such high doses of acid suppressors wipe out nearly all stomach acid secretion, creating a state of chronic achlorhydria. Despite this, only modest, at best, improvement in asthma symptoms is achieved. The implications of this type of treatment are truly frightening. If chronically low acid

---

*Most physicians are required to earn a certain number of CME credits each year to maintain their license or certification. Typically, CME credits are earned by taking "courses" that are offered by mail, online, or live at meetings held at conventions and other locations. It is very common for such courses to be underwritten by pharmaceutical (patent medicine) companies. Although the courses are supposed to be neutral with regard to the promotion of any specific product, and the company is supposed to have no voice in their content, this is a very fuzzy line that is often crossed. For example, the faculty is almost always on the company payroll, and the topic area and approach to the subject are invariably driven by the corporate sponsor's desire to promote its drugs. In many cases, the company influence is even more blatant. As a result, such "educational" programs often turn out to be little more than barely disguised drug promotions that physicians are required to sit through.

secretion can *cause* asthma, as Dr. Bray and others have suggested, isn't it possible that taking these drugs over the course of many years will actually *increase* the risks of asthma in some sensitive people and make them even more dependent on conventional corticosteroid and bronchiodilating drugs? Can such a small improvement in symptoms, if and when it occurs, be worth the potential cost? It's hard to see how this kind of treatment could be justified.

As we will see in chapter 7, there are far better, *natural* ways of reducing acid reflux and relieving asthma that go directly to the causes of these disorders, producing significant improvement without suppressing symptoms and without endangering our health in the process.

Allergies, Food Sensitivities, and Leaky Guts

Over the years, reports have consistently appeared in the medical literature—especially in Europe—linking hypochlorhydria and achlorhydria not just with asthma but with a wide range of allergic reactions and skin disorders. From his vantage point at the Asthma Clinic at the Hospital for Sick Children in London, Dr. George Bray found that asthma was not the only problem in children with low stomach acid. Compared to children with normal stomach acid, they also seemed to have a disproportionate risk of conditions like hay fever, hives, eczema, and migraines.[24] (Dr. Bray also reported that 50 percent of asthmatic parents of asthmatic children had "a definite deficiency of free acid secretion," while the other 50 percent were normal.) Since then, others have also reported associations between low stomach acid and severe acne,[25] chronic hives,[26] dermatitis herpetiformis (a type of skin rash),[27-29] gallbladder disease,[30-31] and hay fever (allergic rhinitis).[32]

How can a deficiency in stomach acid cause us to sneeze, wheeze, or itch? No one knows for sure, but ever since Dr. Bray's day, the answer has been thought to lie in food allergies and sensitivities.

Whether hypochlorhydria causes food allergies or food allergies cause hypochlorhydria is a chicken-and-egg issue. No matter which one sets off the process, a vicious circle soon ensues in which an allergic reaction to food inflames the gastric and intestinal linings, inhibiting HCl secretion and promoting allergic reactions all over the body, not just to foods, but to inhalants and microorganisms, as well.

It is well known that for some sensitive people, inhaling certain allergy-causing substances (*allergens*) like dust, molds, or chemicals can trigger an allergic inflammatory reaction in the airways—an asthmatic attack where the airways become inflamed, swollen, and constricted. Less well recognized is the fact that, for some children, wheezing can often begin with a glass of "Nature's most perfect food," the source of countless celebrity mustaches, good old cow's milk. Thanks to myth, custom, advertising, and political influence, cow's milk is right up there with motherhood and apple pie as an untouchable icon in U.S. society. But the fact is, for quite a large percentage of the population, cow's milk is a poison that can make them very sick. In infants, an allergy to cow's milk is a well-known cause of gastroesophageal reflux.[33–40] There seems to be little doubt that drinking cow's milk can also cause some infants to develop type I diabetes, which can leave them dependent on insulin injections for the rest of their lives.[41–42] When people cannot tolerate cow's milk* (or any other substance), consuming a glassful can cause an inflammatory reaction in the stomach, intestines, or both.

Inflaming the Stomach

When the stomach lining gets inflamed, parietal cells die, and HCl secretion falls off. Finnish investigators found severely impaired gastric acid secretion in eight out of eight cow's milk–intolerant infants, including three who had virtually no HCl in their stomachs. An inflammatory reaction had seriously damaged the infants' gastric mucosal lining, leading to atrophic gastritis (proven with stomach biopsies). After the infants were switched to human or soy milk, their gastric function eventually returned to normal.[43]

As the Finnish study showed, when children continue to drink milk despite the fact that they may be allergic to it, the damage to their stomach lining may be sufficient to cause hypochlorhydria or worse, which impedes the production of pepsin and intrinsic factor. The combination of low acid, low pepsin, and low intrinsic factor impairs the digestion of proteins and the absorption and utilization of vitamin B_{12} (see chapter 4).

Breaching the Intestinal Barrier

Milk or other allergenic proteins that reach the bowels undigested or partially digested due to hypochlorhydria or achlorhydria can trigger an

---

*It is important to distinguish a true milk sensitivity reaction from "lactose intolerance." In lactose intolerance, the immune system is not involved. Instead, the individual cannot tolerate milk because he or she lacks an enzyme required to digest lactose, a primary form of sugar found in milk. When the undigested milk sugar reaches the intestines, it causes nausea, cramps, bloating, gas, and diarrhea.

inflammatory reaction here as well. The resulting damage to the intestinal lining punches holes in one of the body's most important protective barriers, resulting in *intestinal hyperpermeability*, sometimes known as *"leaky gut"* syndrome.[44-47]

Since the GI tract is essentially an extension of the outside world, one of its chief functions is to keep undigested foreign proteins where they belong, in the bowels, but "outside" the body. A healthy intestinal lining allows vitamins, minerals, amino acids, and other products of digestion to pass through its cells and into the general circulation. But it keeps out "foreign" food proteins, bacteria, viruses, fungi, and anything else that might come down the esophagus.

In sensitive people, "foreign" proteins that manage to cross the intestinal barrier and leak into the general circulation can become the object of a vigorous allergic "rejection" reaction by the immune system. We may experience this reaction in range of different ways, from GI discomfort and hives to a potentially fatal generalized "anaphylactic" reaction, in which major systems of the body, including the respiratory tract, begin to break down. Ordinarily, once an allergen is removed, the reaction dissipates. Avoid the allergen and we avoid the reaction.

In some people, though, the picture becomes more complicated, because the initial allergic reaction can somehow trigger the immune system to turn its attack on the body itself. Depending on which part of the body suffers the immune system's misguided attack, a variety of different *autoimmune* diseases can result. These include *rheumatoid arthritis, lupus erythematosus, multiple sclerosis, ulcerative colitis,* and many others. (See below for more about autoimmune diseases.)

Among the most important factors that influence whether or not the intestinal barrier springs a leak is none other than the gastric pH. (This is getting monotonous, isn't it? Gastric pH seems to play important roles all over the GI tract.) In this case, an elevated pH interferes with protein digestion and permits bacterial overgrowth, which combine to promote gut leakage:

- **Impeding protein digestion.** The digestion of protein by pepsin into amino acids occurs most efficiently when the pH in the stomach is less than 3. In the absence of sufficient HCl in the stomach, the pH rises and large amounts of protein go undigested. Instead of the component amino acids passing into the small intestine, whole proteins may slip through.

• **Making the gut leak.** In earlier chapters we described how bacterial overgrowth (due to atrophic gastritis and/or acid-suppressing drugs) can inhibit nutrient absorption and lay the groundwork for stomach cancer. Bacteria may also be the missing link between low gastric acidity and some cases of joint and connective tissue inflammation and other forms of autoimmune disease. For example, people with rheumatoid arthritis often have considerable bacterial overgrowth in their stomachs. It is thought that products of these bacteria may directly damage joints and other tissues, but they may wreak even more havoc when bacterial toxins damage the lining of the small intestine.[48] Such damage can weaken the lining, making it more permeable—or leaky—to proteins and other nutritional molecules that would not normally be permitted to pass through.

Rheumatoid Arthritis and Other Autoimmune Diseases

Rheumatoid arthritis (RA) is a crippling systemic inflammatory disease that affects many different organs, especially the joints. Over time, chronic inflammation can destroy the knee, hip, wrist, and other joints, making movement painful and ultimately impossible. RA is an autoimmune disease. The relationship between RA and digestive functioning may serve as a model for all autoimmune disorders.

In many people, RA begins with a leaky gut. When the gut becomes leaky, no matter what caused it, foreign proteins can slip through the intestinal lining and enter the circulation, where they don't belong. It's not long before they light up the immune system's radar, which responds by scrambling a battalion of proteins called *antibodies*, which are programmed to search out and destroy the invading proteins (*allergens*). The subsequent meeting of the two forces often takes the form of an inflammatory sensitivity or allergic reaction. For some allergens, the battlefield may be the skin (e.g., hives, rashes); for others, the airways (e.g., asthma). It is quite common for the battle to be fought in the GI tract itself, resulting in such diseases as atrophic gastritis, celiac disease, inflammatory bowel disease, ulcerative colitis, and others.[49-53]

If all these antibodies ever did was destroy the invading antigen, we might experience transient discomfort (possibly severe) from an *allergic* reaction until all the antigens were destroyed or neutralized. Then the antibodies would retreat to a neutral corner of the body and wait for the next invasion. However, in certain vulnerable people, under circumstances that are not well understood, antibodies created to attack a specific foreign protein (e.g., cow's milk) sometimes start attacking cells in the body that merely resemble the milk protein, in other words, an autoimmune reaction.

Autoimmune diseases can take many different forms, depending on the tissue involved. These diseases include Goodpasture's syndrome (lung and kidney), Hashimoto's thyroiditis and Graves' disease (thyroid gland), systemic lupus erythematosus (connective tissue), rheumatoid arthritis (joints), scleroderma (skin and connective tissue), glomerulonephritis (kidneys), type 1 diabetes mellitus (pancreas), Sjögren's syndrome (eyes, tear glands, salivary glands, connective tissue, joints), inflammatory bowel disease (the GI tract), multiple sclerosis (nerve tissue), and many others. It is fairly common for people with one type of autoimmune disease to also have symptoms of others, as well.[54]

Whatever form they take, though, autoimmune diseases are usually very serious and notoriously difficult to treat by conventional medicine. Once the body starts mistakenly churning out antibodies against its own tissues, of which there's a virtually endless supply, there's may be no stopping it—at least until all the tissues are gone. That's why autoimmune diseases are such serious business.

Zeroing in on the Wrong Target

Since conventional medicine has never met an inflammatory reaction it didn't try to suppress, the standard treatment for RA (and most other autoimmune diseases) has long been some kind of anti-inflammatory drug. By squelching the inflammatory response (in other words, suppressing part of the immune system), these drugs may achieve a degree of temporary symptomatic relief. Ultimately, though, they always fail, because symptom suppression does nothing to remove the cause or to arrest the progress of the inflammation. If we stop taking the drug, the inflammation comes right back. (Another recurring theme: Recall what happens when you stop taking acid-suppressing drugs—the heartburn comes back, sometimes with a vengeance.)

Anti-inflammatory drugs of all classes have always been dangerous agents with long lists of potential adverse effects, including death. The major anti-inflammatories used to treat RA (and other inflammatory diseases) include:

- **Steroids.** These are among the most powerful anti-inflammatories available. Most steroids are patented or formerly patented synthetic chemical cousins of the natural adrenal steroid hormone, *hydrocortisone* (e.g., Prednisone). They are very dangerous immune suppressors, even when used "as directed."

- **Nonsteroidal anti-inflammatory drugs, or NSAIDs** (e.g., aspirin, Motrin, Advil, and other forms of the drug ibuprofen). Less powerful that the steroids, many of these drugs are available without prescription despite the fact that they can be extremely dangerous, particularly if used for a long time, as they are by people with arthritis. Although NSAIDs are generally considered to be safer than steroids, their use is still associated with seventy-six thousand hospitalizations and seventy-six hundred deaths per *year* in the United States alone, mostly due to damage to the GI tract (e.g., ulcers).[55]

- **COX-2 inhibitors** (e.g., Celebrex, Vioxx). These second-generation NSAIDs are thought to be kinder to the GI tract than traditional NSAIDs, but the jury is still out due to the lack of large-scale, long-term experience. COX-2 inhibitors are known to inhibit the formation of new blood vessels, suggesting that they might interfere with ulcer healing in the stomach.[56]

Gastric Hypoacidity: A Root of RA?

By zeroing in on symptom suppression, conventional medicine has long ignored an intriguing century-old area of research pointing in a totally different direction. According to these studies, the roots of RA (and other autoimmune diseases) may sometimes lie in a deficiency of stomach acid. As far back as 1912, a group of British physicians reported on ten patients with chronic RA, all of whom had below-normal gastric acid levels. In some cases, acid was completely absent. They found that if they could restore the stomach to a more normal condition by essentially putting back what was missing—HCl, pepsin, and other factors—their patients achieved a degree of improvement in their arthritic symptoms.[57]

Results similar to these have persisted across the decades, with most studies emanating from laboratories and clinics outside the United States, especially from Europe, Asia, and South America.[58-63] A 1939 investigation from Germany, for example, found that those RA patients with the worst disease tended to have little or no acid in their stomachs. For some unknown reason, though, stomach acid secretion eventually returned to normal in several of these individuals, and as it did, their swollen joints began to heal.[64] An Italian review in 1945 cited ten other studies, each demonstrating a high rate of hypochlorhydria and achlorhydria in people with RA. In one of these, people with RA were five times more likely to have achlorhydria than normal controls.[65] Experience at Tahoma Clinic confirms the high likelihood of hypochlorhydria and achlorhydria in individuals with RA.

During the 1920s, 1930s, and 1940s, when high-dose aspirin was virtually the only pharmaceutical anti-inflammatory drug available, the connection between gastric acidity and RA was one of the few real leads medicine had into the cause, safe treatment, and possible cure of RA. Beginning in the late 1940s, though, patent medicine companies started bringing out—and heavily promoting—their powerful anti-inflammatory drugs. The quick fix of symptom (inflammation) suppression quickly became established as *the* treatment for RA.

The promising research suggesting the value of investigating and dealing with problems of gastric acidity was unsupported by any patent medicine company money, because no patentable products appeared to be involved, just inexpensive, *unpatentable* natural products, like HCl and pepsin.*

A lack of patent medicine company support usually represents the kiss of death for medical research in this country. The large, well-controlled studies the FDA and medical establishment demand to validate any therapeutic entity are so costly to conduct that only the patent medicine companies themselves (and sometimes the federal government) have deep enough pockets to pay for them. Moreover, small, independent studies of "alternative" treatments, which are usually the only kinds possible, rarely get published in major medical journals or presented at medical conventions, which are sponsored primarily by the patent medicine industry. With the credentials these outlets provide lacking, it is easy for medical authorities—in a perfect example of "catch-22" logic—to dismiss nonpatent medicine research as "unproven" at best or "quackery" at worst.

Thus, it is not surprising that once the anti-inflammatory train left the station, the "gastric acidity connection" to RA was soon forgotten by all but a few physicians and researchers who understood the dead end that cortosteroids, NSAIDs and the other anti-inflammatories represented. Yet the flame continues to burn. As recently as 1986, a group of researchers— from the prestigious Karolinska Institute in Sweden—confirmed the find-

---

*Another promising but neglected area of RA research originated with Dr. Roger Wyburn-Mason, who reported finding a specific amoeba in the joints of all individuals with RA whom he examined. He reported successful treatment of these cases with anti-amoebic therapy. No direct link has been observed between Dr. Wyburn-Mason's amoebae and low stomach acid, but in general it's well known that a principal function of normal stomach acid is killing food and water-borne microorganisms, often the source of amoebic infection. For further information, contact the Rheumatoid Disease Foundation at (615) 799-1002.

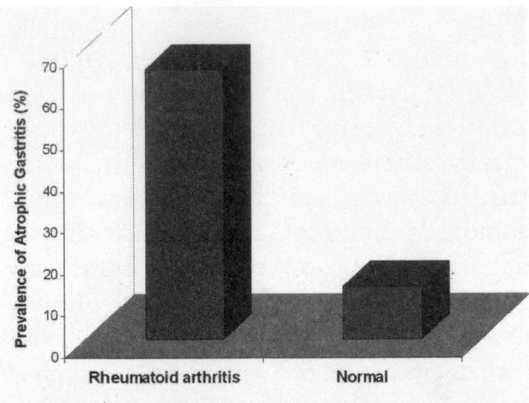

Figure 6-4. People with rheumatoid arthritis have an extremely high rate of atrophic gastritis associated with low stomach acid compared with normal individuals. Adapted from R Marcolongo et al., 1978.

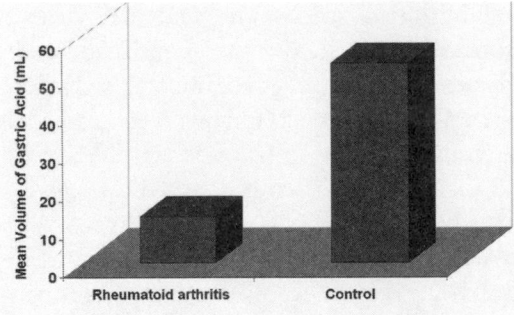

Figure 6-5. Drastically reduced secretion of HCl by the stomachs of people with rheumatoid arthritis. Adapted from Olhagen et al, 1974.

ings of their earlier colleagues.[66] Examining the stomach contents of forty-five RA patients, they found that sixteen (36 percent) had virtually no acid, suggesting they had severe atrophic gastritis. Those people who had suffered from RA the longest had the least acid. Also confirming numerous older studies, the Swedes found that 20 percent of the RA patients they saw had elevated gastrin levels (hypergastrinemia), usually a sign of low stomach acid. Figure 6-4 shows the high rate of atrophic gastritis (65 percent) found in RA patients by a group of Italian researchers.[67] Figure 6-5 shows the results of a British study in which the mean volume of stomach acid secretion was found to be significantly lower in people with RA (and a related form of the disease).[68]

Opening the Door to Autoimmune Diseases

Although NSAIDs (and other anti-inflammatory drugs) are supposed to improve life for RA patients, they are particularly dangerous in the long run, first, because they are so likely to cause GI distress, and second, because they are so widely promoted and so easy to get. Like food allergens, NSAIDs can injure the intestinal lining, causing it to leak.[69–71] And a leaky gut, whether caused by achlorhydria, bacterial infection, food allergy, excessive alcohol, drug reaction, or other causes, may open the door to all kinds of allergic and autoimmune diseases.

Gallstones, Gastric Secretion, and Food Allergies

The gallbladder stores bile, which is produced in the liver, and releases it to aid in the digestion and absorption of fats and other nutrients. Many people develop "stones" in the gallbladder, which can block the flow of bile, causing the gallbladder to become inflamed or infected, oftennecessitating surgery. In addition to recurring abdominal pain, gallstones are also associated with bloating, belching, heartburn, and gas.

Numerous studies dating back to the early 1900s have linked gallbladder disease with low stomach acid secretion.[72] For example, in one study of fifty patients with gallstones, twenty-six had below-normal stomach acid output.[73] Does low stomach acid cause gallbladder disease? Or are both the result of a common cause?

There is very good reason to believe that in most cases of gallstones, the symptoms are the result of food allergy. When sixty-nine people with gallstones were placed on an elimination diet* for a week, every one of them experienced symptom relief. As the foods were added back one by one, the symptoms often returned. It has been hypothesized that food allergy causes the bile ducts to swell, restricting the flow of bile from the gallbladder and promoting the formation of stones.[74]

Can Avoiding Food Allergens Lead to Improvement in People with Autoimmune and Other Related Diseases?

Absolutely so! At Tahoma Clinic and throughout the "natural medicine" world, a mainstay of *any* autoimmune disease treatment program is the identification, elimination, and desensitization of food (and other) allergies and sensitivities. Although this step alone rarely cures autoimmune diseases outright, the improvements achieved are frequently major. No matter what the specific autoimmune problem (please review the list at the beginning of this chapter), working with food allergy is always a major tool.

Similarly, another mainstay of treatment for *any* autoimmune disease is the examination for and (when found) treatment of low stomach acid and other digestive malfunction. Low stomach acid is so common in *any* autoimmune condition that we're surprised when we *don't* find it. Correcting the low stomach acid or other digestive malfunction can also result in major improvement in the autoimmune disease. Although "natu-

---

*In an allergy-elimination diet, likely offending foods are removed from the diet for a period of time and gradually added back in to see which stimulate a reaction.

ral medicine" doctors see improvement achieved repeatedly by following this lead, practitioners of conventional medicine rarely if ever look for low stomach acid and poor digestion in those with autoimmune disease.

Unfortunately, only a handful of small studies have systematically examined the food allergy and autoimmune disease connection, but the results indicate that some people can benefit. For example, in one study, twenty-two people with RA followed an allergy-elimination diet. Arthritis improved for twenty (91 percent) of these people, and nineteen were able to identify specific foods that made them worse.[75] Several other small studies also report favorable responses associated with changes in diet in some people with RA.[76-79] In RA, Alan Gaby, M.D., reports that avoiding allergenic foods works best in younger women (aged twenty-five to forty years) who have less severe cases. He notes that he has seen about fifteen patients who fit that description, and every one of them improved dramatically with only dietary changes.[80]

With lupus, the support is similarly sketchy, but still suggestive. In one report, physicians examining a child diagnosed with lupus found him to have antibodies to milk in his blood. This suggested that his immune system was reacting against milk protein. When milk was removed from the child's diet, his lupus symptoms resolved. On two subsequent occasions when he drank milk, they returned.[81] An Australian study of four people with lupus also found marked improvement in symptoms when they avoided allergenic foods and took certain nutritional supplements. Standard tests used to diagnose and monitor lupus showed these individuals to be normal.[82]

Much more work needs to be done to identify which people are most likely to benefit and to develop ever more effective treatment strategies. Clearly, such research will not come from the pharmaceutical industry, which has long demonstrated its interest only in patentable therapies that do little more than suppress symptoms.

Wouldn't it make much more sense, therapeutically speaking, to try to repair a leaky gut or, better yet, keep it from springing a leak in the first place? To remove the drugs and allergenic foods that may be irritating the GI tract, and possibly triggering dangerous autoimmune reactions? To restore missing stomach acid that would quickly destroy colonizing bacteria and also (along with pepsin) break down proteins before they can leak out into the general circulation?

Restoring the GI tract to a normal, healthy state so that bacteria don't grow in the stomach and foreign proteins don't leak out across the intestinal barrier requires no expensive, dangerous drugs. It can often be accomplished safely and effectively with a variety of natural—*unpatentable*—substances.

Because there are no profits to be made from selling these natural treatments, the pharmaceutical industry, which controls the vast majority of medical research in the United States, will never investigate them or manufacture them. In fact, they will do everything possible to disparage them, because, should the word get out that they exist, natural treatments could threaten their stranglehold on the practice of medicine.

One might ask, if the possibilities of these natural treatments are so good, why isn't the FDA sponsoring or promoting research? Again, the answer is simple. The FDA and the patent medicine industry are two sides of the same coin. The FDA's role has never been to advance the science of medicine. It has no interest in finding a cure for lupus or any other disease. Instead, its role assigned by Congress is to make sure the drugs and foods that get marketed in the United States are safe and effective.

To this end, the FDA has set up a drug approval process that is so expensive and so onerous that it virtually guarantees that only the patent medicine companies can afford to develop new treatments and get them "approved." Thanks to this system, natural treatments, no matter how effective or how safe they may be, are forever destined to carry the label "unproven," as far as the FDA and the medical establishment are concerned. At best an "unproven" treatment may be viewed as harmless and a waste of money. At worst, it may be deemed "dangerous" and the stuff of "quacks." The fact is, without sufficient research, they'll never know what it is really, and that seems to be fine with them.

To those of us who use these treatments every day and who know how safe and effective they can be, using them is, as they say, a "no-brainer." Every day, our patients with "incurable" chronic diseases achieve remarkable relief, and often cures, using nothing more than a carefully selected and carefully applied arsenal of natural therapies. In the next chapter, we will discuss the possibilities of natural treatments for GI and GI-related disorders.

CHAPTER 7
Treating Heartburn and "Acid Indigestion" the Natural Way

"I still can't believe it!" Jon Hitchcock exclaimed. "Taking hydrochloric acid capsules makes my heartburn and 'acid indigestion' go away! Would you tell me how that works, again?"

Before I could answer, his wife, Sara, said: "Don't you remember, Jon? The doctor told you last time . . . after you had your stomach acid measured. No one knows how it works, but for over one hundred years, doctors have observed that bringing low stomach acid towards normal frequently eliminates heartburn, stomach bloating, indigestion? Maybe we should talk about something for your memory."

"But it's just so hard to believe," Jon answered. "For the last ten years, doctors have been telling me I have too much stomach acid, which causes me 'acid indigestion' and 'acid reflux.' They've been prescribing antacids and acid blockers and telling me I'd better stay on them even when my symptoms aren't particularly bad, because 'all that acid' might permanently damage my esophagus. Are you sure taking those hydrochloric acid capsules won't burn my esophagus?"

"Do you feel any burning?" I asked.

"Jon told me he hasn't had any heartburn after meals since the second week he started taking them," Sara observed.

"That's true," Jon said. "But I'd still like to understand. Not just the doctors, but all those TV commercials, all of them telling us about 'hyperacidity' and even showing cartoons of 'acid attacks' on the esophagus. I wouldn't have believed it if I actually hadn't had my own stomach acid measured."

"I'm glad you did," I said. "After looking at literally thousands of very precisely measured stomach acid tests, I've observed that more than nine out of ten of us who suffer from so-called 'acid indigestion' actually have *lack-of-acid* indigestion. Replacing some or all of the missing acid . . . along with the stomach enzyme pepsin . . . eliminates heartburn, gas, bloating and indigestion in most cases."

"But I'd still like to understand how it works," Jon said. "I'm an engineer. It bugs me not knowing. If I hadn't seen the measurement on my own stomach, I wouldn't even have tried that betaine hydrochloride-pepsin stuff."

"I'm sorry I don't have an explanation for how it works," I said. "With enough research money, I'm sure it could be figured out, but there's no money in researching natural, unpatentable remedies. So for now, we just go with observed results."

Jon smiled. "I have to admit that engineering isn't a 100 percent exact science at all times, either. We engineers like to maintain the public illusion, though. But we are a lot more exact than medicine appears to be. Nearly ten years of diagnosing 'overacidity,' and no one *actually measured* my stomach acid."

"I'm glad Sara persuaded you." I paused for a moment. "You're an engineer. How about an engineering theory? Unproven, of course."

"Why not? A theory's better than no answer at all."

"How about a feedback loop theory?"

"That's basic engineering. Tell me about it."

"Hope you have a few minutes."

"Long as you don't charge extra." Jon smiled.

"I won't, I promise. OK . . . What you've seen on TV and heard from doctors is partly true. Heartburn pain is caused by acid, but not *too much* acid. Even though there's actually too little acid, even a small amount in the wrong place, the esophagus, can really hurt. Remember, acid doesn't burn a normal stomach. Our stomachs are built to withstand acid, to *produce* acid, acid as much as one-hundred-thousand times stronger than normal tissue acidity. Acid of that strength is absolutely necessary for optimal digestion.

"By contrast, our esophaguses . . . esophagi? . . . whatever . . . aren't built to handle any acid at all, not even weak acid. So under normal circumstances, the esophagus is protected against acid reflux by a circular muscle called the lower esophageal sphincter. When functioning normally, the sphincter opens to allow food and liquids to drop through, and closes to prevent stomach acid from refluxing back up into the esophagus.

"A number of things cause the lower esophageal sphincter to malfunction and lose its ability to close when it should. Nicotine and caffeine are common offenders. Alcohol does it for some. Unrecognized food allergies and sensitivities are a much more common cause of lower esophageal sphincter malfunction than is usually recognized. But in my experience, low stomach acid is the most common cause.

"Now I'll get to that 'feedback loop' theory. Let's see . . . I know, you're an engineer, but I don't think Sara is, so . . . I know." I turned to Sara. "Ever taken the top off the back of the toilet?"

Sara looked surprised. "Yes."

"I'm sure you noticed water rushing in when the tank's empty. As the water level rises, it lifts a float, which activates a valve, which slowly turns down the water inflow until it shuts off." I turned back to Jon. "I realize that's an imperfect analogy from a mechanical system, but it's close. It's quite possible, although not proven, that as the acid level rises . . . technically, the pH level drops . . . that a normally functioning lower esophageal sphincter (or a tissue close to it) 'senses' the increasing acidity, and shuts itself. Briefly put, an 'acid-sensitive feedback loop' leading to sphincter muscle closure. But it's just a theory, no proof, and reality may be something else."

Jon thought for a moment. "Sounds reasonable. But no one's checked this out?"

"Not that I . . . we . . . can find. What I mean by that is, I've looked, and some very able young doctors have spent hours in medical libraries looking, but we can't find any research on the point."

"Well, I'll just take the practical engineering point of view and agree that my experience . . . like yours . . . shows that taking hydrochloric acid in capsules shuts off acid reflux into my esophagus," Jon said. "The next question is: I'm forty-nine. Will I need to take hydrochloric acid-pepsin capsules with meals for the next forty-nine years, should I live so long?"

"You're more likely to have those next forty-nine years if you do," Sara said. "That's why I nagged you to come in here to get tested in the first place! Don't you remember . . . we really do need something for his memory, Doctor," she smiled. "Don't you remember I told you that if you kept taking those acid blockers, you wouldn't be digesting your protein properly, you wouldn't be getting all the amino acids from it that you should? You wouldn't be digesting and absorbing minerals as well as possible. I've noticed you have a little bit more energy, a bit more 'get up and go' in just the short time since you've started normalizing your digestion. You just can't live as long or as healthy if you're not getting your nutrition!"

"Sara's right," I agreed. "And all that enthusiasm shows she cares, too. But to answer your question . . . although it's harder to do as we get older, a few of us do get our stomachs back to fully normal, acid-producing function. It doesn't 'just happen' though. It usually takes working on it, on purpose."

"How?"

"There are two basic aspects: Removing 'bad stuff' that interferes with normal function, and using 'good stuff' and other techniques to encourage normal function. Included on the 'bad stuff' side is checking for the stomach bacteria *Helicobacter pylori*—we checked you for that, it was negative—and getting rid of it when it's found. Other 'bad stuff' for normal stomach function includes food allergies for many of us, especially to milk and dairy products. It's been proven that in some cases, food allergy or sensitivity can seriously interfere with normal function. For infants, it's absolutely nailed down that cow's milk causes gastroesophageal reflux, and removing cow's milk eliminates the problem."

"How about reflux in adults?"

"I've found food allergy, especially cow's milk and dairy allergy, to be a frequent cause of, or contributor to, gastroesophageal reflux in many adults, but unfortunately no one's published 'controlled' research. Now, where were we? Oh yes . . . it's also best to eliminate refined sugar, because it's a direct stomach irritant. I know you don't smoke, but if you did, I'd recommend you stop."

"What about alcohol?"

"Beer and wine don't appear to be a problem, especially wine. There may even be something to the adage that a little wine with meals improves the digestion, though it's not proven. But distilled, higher-proof alcohol is definitely a no-no. High-proof alcohol is actually a good way to 'pickle' or abnormally preserve tissue.

"But that's not all. Fluoride and chlorine in the water can inhibit one or more of the enzymes that our stomachs use to make acid, so even though there are only very small quantities of either one in most municipal water, it's best to drink water with no chlorine or fluoride content.

"Now, the 'good stuff' side. For literally centuries, in many European countries, older folks have drunk 'bitters' before meals to improve digestive function. Bitter drinks taken before meals are called 'aperitifs.' In the early 1900s, one researcher claimed that bitters didn't help digestion, but others found that bitters actually increase stomach secretion of hydrochloric acid and pepsin if digestive secretion is below optimum to begin with, if the bitters are actually tasted—they don't work if they're swallowed without being tasted—and there must be food in the stomach for them to work."

"That all makes engineering sense. No point having them work if there's nothing in the stomach to work on, or if the stomach is working OK anyway."

"More modern research has supported the earlier work. Liquid preparations of both gentian and artemisia—two of the most commonly used bitters preparations—taken five minutes before meals, stimulate secretion of digestive juices. Both liquid herbals also improve bile flow from the liver, and that helps digestion, too, although at a later stage."

"So if I decide to use them, what do I do?"

"Find a liquid preparation of gentian or artemisia . . . it's also called wormwood. A usual dose is five to ten drops of a one-to-five dilution in about twenty milliliters—that's about one and one-half tablespoonsful—of water, taken about fifteen minutes before meals. Most herbalists recommend that bitters-in-water be sipped slowly."

"I'm glad you're writing that down."

"Sorry, I know it's a bit technical. Your natural food store or compounding pharmacy can help you with this, too."

"Anything else I can do to try to get my stomach function back to normal on its own?"

"Nothing else is specifically known at the present time. As I mentioned, there's no financial incentive for research on the point. Just do everything you can to improve your health in general: good diet, supplements, exercise . . . "

"You forgot two things, doctor," Sara said.

"Tell us."

"Well, you didn't really forget one of them, but I know Jon , it really needs to be reemphasized. He's not been a very good supplement taker, but he's *got* to remember to take his betaine hydrochloride-pepsin capsules with *every* meal! Not only will they help him digest and absorb all his nutrients better, but they're also essential to his chances of digesting and absorbing all the nutrients his stomach needs to repair itself!" She looked at Jon.

Jon threw up his hands. "OK, OK, I got it, Sara. I'll be good."

"I'm not just picking on you, Jon. I've read in any number of places that if we live long enough, we're very likely to have our digestion get weak. So I expect to need to take digestive aids someday, too."

"And what's the second thing?" Jon asked Sara.

"Prayer, visualization, meditation—techniques to focus your *intention* to improve your health, in this case your stomach."

"What about those, Doctor?" Jon asked.

"You picked a very wise woman to marry," I replied.

• • •

Acid neutralization and/or suppression *seem* like they ought to be good ways to treat heartburn/GERD/ "acid indigestion" . . . as long as we pretend that these conditions are caused by too much stomach acid and that, although the body goes to great lengths to concentrate HCl only in the stomach, it doesn't really need it. The vast majority of Americans—physicians and nonphysicians alike—urged on by a pharmaceutical industry raking in more than $7 billion a year in anti-acid product sales, understandably chooses to believe these myths. They minimize the risks associated with bacterial overgrowth, and they deny the value of HCl for protein digestion. As one prominent introductory medical textbook, *A Digest of Digestion*, states quite clearly: "Acid and pepsin are *not* essential for protein digestion." The author posits that pancreatic enzymes are sufficient to do the job.

He is wrong, of course. He completely ignores the effect of acid on mineral digestion and absorption. He offers no proof from controlled studies that protein digestion and subsequent amino acid and peptide absorption is the same with or without stomach acid. He neglects to mention that pancreatic enzyme secretion may be impaired in states of hypochlorhydria and achlorhydria (remember the "digestive cascade"?). But because this view is taught in most medical schools, young doctors soon learn to ignore the value of HCl and pepsin for proper digestion. They forget about the bacterial barrier stomach acid provides. The only time acid seems to come up on their radar is when it's "causing" an ulcer, heartburn, GERD, or esophageal cancer. As a result, acid has come to be vilified as something to be feared and suppressed the minute it appears to start causing trouble, and sometimes before.

If stomach acid is causing pain or discomfort, then it follows that the less we've got of it, the better. If Tums or Rolaids isn't doing the job, then why not roll out one of the big guns, like Pepcid or Zantac, or better yet, Prilosec or Prevacid, and drive a stake through the acid monster's heart? In fact, the trend today, as evidenced by the widespread promotion and sky-rocketing sales of powerful acid-blocking drugs, is to go after even the mildest cases of heartburn with these gastrointestinal "nuclear weapons." Hard as it is to believe, the manufacturers of Prilosec recently asked the FDA to allow them to sell their drug over the counter.* Fortunately, in a rare moment of sanity, an FDA advisory panel turned them down, at least for now.

As we have been suggesting throughout this book, there is a better way to deal with "acid indigestion," a natural way, a way that works *with* the body's physiology, not against it. We believe, and much of the scientific evidence—not to mention common sense—supports us, that stomach acid is there for a reason (several reasons, really) and that when the flames of so-called acid indigestion start to erupt, it's more likely a reflection of *too little acid*, not too much.

Thus, the only treatment strategy that makes any sense is to give the GI tract back what it's missing, not deplete it further. If HCl is low, replace it with HCl; likewise for pepsin and other digestive enzymes. Not only does this strategy work to eliminate heartburn and GERD, it often goes a long way toward restoring any nutrient deficiencies and repairing the gastric bacterial barrier, not to mention the intestinal barrier.

Since the GI system never has a drug deficiency, no drugs are necessary to restore it to its normal state. Everything we recommend in the following pages is either a natural constituent of the GI system, like HCl and pepsin, or else a naturally occurring substance, like licorice or mastic, that helps heal by restoring the normal state but has little or no propensity for causing harm when used as directed.

In cases of mild to moderate heartburn, "acid indigestion," bloating, and gas, actual testing for stomach acid production at Tahoma Clinic (see page 133) shows that hypochlorhydria (too little acid production) occurs in over 90 percent of thousands tested since 1976. In these cases, a "natural strategy" is almost always successful.

Even in severe cases diagnosed as GERD, actual testing also shows hypochlorhydria in over 90 percent of cases. Unfortunately, when the problem is severe, particularly when there's tissue damage in the esopha-

---

*It's not hard to believe from the manufacturer's point of view, though. With its patent about to run out and with even more powerful drugs coming down the pipeline, Prilosec is a perfect candidate to join Zantac, Pepcid, and the other "has-been" acid suppressors on drug store and supermarket shelves—a truly chilling prospect!

gus, it may be too late for an entirely natural strategy. Under these circumstances, we recommend the relatively new surgical procedures such as "gastroplication," which repairs the LES valve. These procedures do not have the potential to create nutrient deficiencies and disease the way acid blockers do. However, even some severe cases of GERD can be gradually brought back under control with natural means.

In more severe cases, it's *very important* to work with a physician who is skilled and knowledgeable in nutritional medicine. Also, since there are (very rare) possible adverse effects from the use of hydrochloric acid-pepsin capsules, it's best to work with such a physician whenever using this material.

Understandably, conventional medicine looks askance at such a natural approach, scoffing at the strange "drugs" it endorses and the apparent lack of research support. From this point of view, its basic premise, treating so-called "acid indigestion" with *acid* (and other natural techniques), seems patently absurd.

And while we're on the subject of patents, let's not lose sight of the fact that all these natural treatments are *unpatentable*. As we've pointed out numerous times in this book, patent medicine companies, which control most of the medical research in this country, are interested only in patented "proprietary" products, which only they can sell. By definition, that excludes *all natural products*, which cannot be patented. Not only do they have no interest in developing them, they have every reason to disparage them, because they represent safe, effective, inexpensive competition.

Many journal articles and textbooks purporting to systematically examine HCl replacement have reached decidedly negative conclusions regarding natural treatments. In one typical "legitimate" study, published in the *New England Journal of Medicine*, the author concluded that, in cases where people had no measurable stomach acid, " . . . treatment with a bland diet, sedation, and adequate attention to colonic evacuation appears to be more efficacious than substitution [HCl] therapy."[1]

Yet, a close reading of this study reveals serious flaws. For example, the author noted that, in people treated with HCl, heartburn symptoms actually diminished early in the treatment, only to return later, even though the treatment was unchanged. Instead of seeing the glass half full here, the author chose to see it half empty, using this finding to argue that replacing acid makes no difference. However, he replaced only a small quantity of HCl, despite the fact that his test subjects had serious achlorhydria and could also be assumed to be deficient in pepsin activity and vitamin B_{12} absorption. Those of us who treat "acid indigestion" successfully every day using natural remedies know that acid replacement usually works best when adequate acid replacement is used and pepsin and vitamin B_{12} are also restored. Nor did the researcher add calcium or iron to his test subjects' diets, despite the fact that these minerals are not well-absorbed by people with low stomach acid. And despite the fact that in some cases symptoms were admittedly "provoked by specific food groups," he *did not* recommend elimination of those foods for the duration of the HCl treatment.

Is it any surprise the conclusions were so negative? As we have described throughout this book, the use of HCl for treating various disorders related to GI dysfunction has a long history that predates the modern pharmaceutical industry. While many of the early studies may not stand up to some of the rigorous design criteria demanded by today's prospective, double-blind, placebo-controlled standards, some do hold up quite well. Moreover, we should remember that the early researchers were not driven primarily by the desire to sell products. Large investigational grants—such as those offered by the patent medicine industry—were unknown in those days. Medical research tended to be less formal, more personal, and often less biased. For the most part, the early investigators were dedicated, careful observers who conducted small-scale studies on patients in their own clinics or hospitals. With no built-in commercial bias, their findings have shown consistent benefits of HCl/pepsin/vitamin B_{12} replacement with hardly any serious adverse effects. There are simply too many examples to dismiss all the findings because they are "anecdotal" or from "poorly controlled" studies.

While large, well-controlled trials are certainly desirable, they are not the only pathway to scientific truth, especially if they are serving a commercial purpose as well as a scientific one. Biased results and conflicts of interest in pharmaceutically sponsored research—despite the fact that studies are usually technically "well controlled"—are becoming a major bone of contention in American medicine. Recent editorials in both the *Journal of the American Medical Association*[2-3] and the *New England Journal of Medicine*,[4-5] the two most prestigious and influential general medical publications in the United States, have decried the increasing influence of marketing pressures on the direction of medical research and, by implication, medical practice.

One of the earliest but still applicable definitions of "science" is close observation of Nature. Consider this bit of "common sense" observation: Why would Nature expend so much metabolic energy to provide each one of us *at birth* (and until at least age forty) with an ample supply of stomach acid and pepsin if it weren't really necessary for digestion? It's easy to see the harm that hypochlorhydria and achlorhydria can cause, if we know enough to look for it. It's also easy to see remarkable recoveries from illnesses usually deemed chronic, incurable, or both, using the natural treatments and techniques described in this chapter. It is unfortunate that most physicians today are looking in the wrong direction when it comes to gastrointestinal health.

What's Actually Going On in the Stomach?

When patients come to the Tahoma Clinic with GI distress (or one of the many diseases that may be related to GI dysfunction, or, very likely, both), one of the first things we do is try to find out how well their stomachs are working by measuring their gastric pH. While this measure, known as *gastric analysis*, would seem to be an obvious first step, it is rarely used in conventional medical practice, even in cases of GERD, when *hyper*acidity is often presumed.

Gastric analysis has a long history in medicine, going back at least to the early nineteenth century. In most cases, the gastric contents were sampled through a slender tube that was passed into the stomach. Once pumped out of the stomach, the gastric juice could then be analyzed and its pH measured. Although this technique can provide useful information regarding the pH and the composition of the gastric juice, it has obvious limitations in everyday practice.

In fact, measuring the stomach's acid-secreting capacity can be quite simple. We use a device called a Heidelberg capsule, which consists of a tiny pH sensor and a radio transmitter compressed into something that resembles a large vitamin capsule.[6-7]

Although it sounds like a modern computerized instrument, variations of the Heidelberg capsule have actually been around since the 1960s. When swallowed, the sensors in the capsule measure the pH of the stomach contents and relay the findings by radio signal to a receiver located outside the body. A computer and printer connected to the receiver records a continuous record of gastric pH for as long as the capsule remains in the stomach (which can be several hours without much discomfort). Since the capsule is tethered to a long thread, it can be easily removed from the stomach once the test is completed. (Heidelberg capsules without tethers are sometimes used to evaluate the entire GI tract.)

In a typical gastric analysis, after swallowing the capsule, the individual being tested ingests a solution of baking soda, which turns the gastric juice alkaline. As the stomach lining continues to secrete HCl, the pH gradually falls back into the acidic range. The rate at which the pH changes from alkaline back to acidic through a series of bicarbonate challenges provides a very accurate measurement of the stomach's ability to produce HCl.

Stomach acidity can also be estimated indirectly by analyzing samples of hair for mineral content. If the hair is deficient in a large majority of minerals, particularly those known to be poorly absorbed in low acid states (e.g., iron, calcium, zinc), gastric hypochlorhydria or achlorhydria is a strong possibility. This method is not nearly as accurate or as definitive as a Heidelberg capsule, but it may provide useful information, especially for young children who cannot swallow a capsule.

The use of acid-suppressing or acid-neutralizing medications *presumes* an excess of HCl in the stomach, but most physicians never know what the state of acid secretion is in the stomach, because they never look. In some cases, they might measure *esophageal* pH, but as we have noted earlier, this tells us nothing about what's going on in the stomach. It can only confirm that acid has indeed refluxed into the esophagus.

Physicians who actually measure gastric acidity in their heartburn/GERD patients often find that the pH is higher than it should be (higher pH = less acid = relatively alkaline). If most physicians did this, perhaps they would think twice about prescribing drugs that suppress acid secretion further.

Reducing Reflux via Dietary and Lifestyle Changes

Gastroesophageal reflux happens for a lot of reasons. Acid secretion can be low, high, or normal. The common thread that runs through virtually all cases is an LES valve that allows the stomach contents to back up into the esophagus. The reason the LES isn't doing its job can often be traced to the things we eat, drink, or smoke; to the drugs we take; and sometimes to our level of stress. The following factors can all weaken the LES, directly irritate the esophageal lining, or simply force acidic gastric juice back up through the LES into the esophagus:

- Some foods, including fats, chocolate, coffee, mints (especially peppermint and spearmint), sugar, onions, and some alcoholic beverages, can weaken the LES, making it more likely to open inappropriately (TLESRs).

- Other foods, including acidic citrus fruits and tomato-based foods, spicy foods, carbonated beverages, and coffee, can further irritate an already inflamed esophageal lining.

- Remember the series of research studies cited in the last chapter proving that cow's milk causes gastroesophageal reflux in infants? Many *adults* observe that reflux is lessened or even disappears when food allergens (especially cow's milk and dairy, but many others, too) are eliminated.

- Because a large volume of food in the stomach can increase the frequency of TLESRs, overeating can cause reflux. Sufficient volume and/or pressure of gas will also force the stomach contents through the LES.

- Certain medications can weaken the LES. These include bronchodilators used to treat asthma (e.g., theophylline, albuterol, ephedrine), NSAIDs, certain types of blood-pressure-lowering drugs (e.g., calcium channel blockers, beta-blockers), the antianxiety drug Valium, the narcotic analgesic Demerol, and nitroglycerine (and related drugs) used to treat coronary artery disease (angina). These drugs all function, in one way or another, to relax muscles, including those that surround the airways and blood vessels, but also those that comprise much of the GI tract.

- Some medications can directly irritate the gastrointestinal lining, leading to heartburn, esophageal and peptic ulcers, and leaky gut. These drugs include aspirin, NSAIDs (e.g., ibuprofen, naproxen, and many others), the antibiotic tetracycline, the cardiac antiarrhythmic drug quinidine, potassium chloride tablets, and iron salts. GI irritation is a major side effect of some of these drugs, causing great injury and severely limiting their use.

- Activities such as coughing, wheezing, bending from the waist, heavy lifting, straining at stool, and certain types of exercise can all increase intra-abdominal pressure. The increased pressure can literally force the stomach contents through the LES, especially if the stomach is full and/or the LES is already weakened. Heartburn is so much more common in pregnancy because the growing fetus compresses the entire upper GI tract.

- Gravity can also play an important role. Reflux is far more likely when we lie on our backs or sides than when we stand upright, which is one reason why most serious reflux events occur during sleep. When we stand, gravity helps draw the stomach contents away from the LES, but when we are reclining, stomach contents tend to remain in the upper portion of the stomach.

Once we are aware of which factors might be triggering our heartburn, eliminating them may be all that is required to relieve or prevent reflux. Of course, breaking certain long-standing food and drug habits may not be easy. Nevertheless, understanding the health benefits that can accrue from elimination—including heartburn relief, reducing the risks associated with GERD, elimination of acid-suppressing drugs, return of normal gastric function, improved nutrient absorption, better health, and longer life—may provide a little extra motivation.

Avoid These Foods and Drugs That Can Cause Heartburn

LES Weakeners	Esophageal Irritants
Foods • Fats • Chocolate • Coffee • Mints, especially peppermint and spearmint • Sugar • Alcohol • Onions • Food allergies **Drugs** • Cigarettes • Bronchodilators (e.g., theophylline, albuterol, ephedrine) • NSAIDs • Calcium channel blockers (e.g., Cardizem, many others) • Beta-blockers (e.g., Inderal, many others) • Diazepam (Valium) • Nitrates (e.g., nitroglycerin) • Demerol	**Foods** • Citrus fruits and juices • Tomato-based foods • Spicy foods • Coffee • Carbonated drinks **Drugs** • Aspirin • NSAIDs • Tetracycline • Quinidine • Potassium chloride tablets • Iron salts

First Steps: Heading Off Heartburn at Home

The diet and lifestyle changes listed below can often be extremely effective all by themselves in reducing and preventing reflux. For example, elevating the head of the bed by six inches in order to allow gravity to help keep the gastric contents away from the LES is almost as effective for healing reflux esophagitis as taking Zantac.[8]

However, no matter what other herbal (or drug) treatments are implemented, they should always be *in addition* to these dietary and lifestyle changes, not instead of them. It makes no sense to use drugs or natural treatments on the one hand and then turn around and eat foods, take drugs, and do other things that promote reflux on the other.

- Avoid the foods and drugs shown in the table on page 136. (Food allergies will, of course, vary from individual to individual.)

- Eat smaller meals.

- Minimize activity that might increase intra-abdominal pressure, for example, bending or heavy lifting.

- Wear loose-fitting clothing that does not squeeze the abdomen and put added pressure on the LES.

- Limit food intake (especially the foods in the table on page 136) during the hours just prior to bedtime.

- Elevate the head of the bed using four- to eight-inch blocks.

It is regrettable that the marketers of anti-acid products are putting out the message in their advertising that we can have our burrito and eat it, too. All we need to do is pop a Pepcid or a Prilosec first or a Tums or Maalox afterward. And the physicians who prescribe these products, possibly in very high doses to people with "intractable" heartburn, generally make little effort to get their patients to alter any possibly self-destructive behaviors. Most people who buy these products off the shelf are going to feel that using them is all they need to do to rid themselves of "acid indigestion." While some doctors may suggest changes in diet or behavior and/or hand out brochures outlining the steps listed above along with their prescriptions, it's always much easier—for both doctor and patient—to just prescribe a pill. This is especially true when the patient, primed by the flood of patent medicine company ads, comes in demanding a prescription. Does anybody ever give a second thought to the potential consequences of profound, chronic gastric acid suppression? We sincerely doubt it.

Replacing HCl and Pepsin

Paradoxical as it may seem to those schooled in pharmaceutical medicine, replacing HCl in people with hypochlorhydria or achlorhydria can be a very effective way of eliminating heartburn/indigestion/GERD and other GI symptoms, not to mention the many diseases linked to low stomach acidity.

When I treat patients with HCl, I always make clear that while it can be extremely effective, it is not without its risks, and is, therefore, not for everyone:*

- HCl should only be taken by people who have lower-than-normal gastric acid secretion, as determined by an objective measure, such as gastric analysis.

- Problems related to supplementary HCl are rare, but they can be serious. People taking HCl should be carefully supervised by a physician knowledgeable in its use.

- HCl should never be taken by anyone who is also using any kind of anti-inflammatory medication such as corticosteroids (e.g., Prednisone), aspirin, Indocin, ibuprofen (e.g., Motrin, Advil), or other NSAIDs. These drugs can initiate damage to the GI lining that supplementary HCl might aggravate, increasing the risk of gastric bleeding or ulcer.

- HCl should usually be taken along with pepsin. It is presumed that stomachs that don't produce enough HCl also don't make enough pepsin. Although this presumption has rarely been tested, I have found that HCl replacement usually works better with pepsin than

---

*There are occasions when the risks related to HCl replacement may be higher than we would like. In these cases, as long as the potential benefits outweigh the risks, I may still recommend the treatment. However, before starting, I always explain the possible risks, benefits, and precautions. Once patients start on HCl, I always carefully monitor the course of therapy.

without it. There are rare individuals who are sensitive to pepsin, and they should avoid taking it.

Liquid, Tablets, or Capsules?

Although liquid HCl, which was used back in the early days of replacement therapy, can still be found, it is just what it sounds like, concentrated acid in a bottle, just like we played with in high school chem lab. It is very dangerous stuff and is available for internal use in humans only by prescription. Liquid HCl must be handled very carefully. It is difficult to transport and extremely dangerous if the bottle should break or spill.

"Modern" replacement HCl usually comes in more manageable forms attached to a "carrier," either *betaine* or *glutamic* acid. Attaching the HCl to a carrier yields a powder—*betaine hydrochloride* or *glutamic acid hydrochloride*—that can be contained in a capsule. Typically these products are sold in health food stores and compounding pharmacies, combined with pepsin.

My preference is for the capsule form of HCl. When we compare stool specimens from people who have taken an adequate number of HCl capsules to those who take dilute liquid HCL, capsule use leaves far less undigested material. This suggests that the people taking the capsules are digesting protein more completely. In some people taking the maximum dose of HCl in liquid form, meat may still go virtually undigested. But when they switch to the capsule form, meat (and other protein) digestion immediately improves. In addition, the capsules are safer to handle and produce fewer unwanted side effects.

There's no way to know which form—betaine or glutamic acid HCl—is best suited for a given person. I generally find that if one form causes any side effects, it is worthwhile trying the other, since it's rare that people are sensitive to both forms. However, since the betaine molecule is smaller than the glutamic acid molecule, more HCl can be concentrated in betaine capsules of identical size.

To minimize side effects, it is always best to start with one capsule of betaine HCl containing about 650 mg, with pepsin, in the early part of each meal. If there are no problems after two or three days, I recommend increasing the dose to two capsules in the early part of each meal; then after another two to three days, increase it again to three capsules. We increase the dose gradually in this stepwise fashion until the recommended dose (five to seven capsules for the "average" adult) is reached. When people have to take several capsules with a meal, I suggest taking half just after the first few bites and half midway through the meal.

The most effective adult dose of betaine HCl is 5 to 7 of the 650 milligram capsules per meal, with pepsin. (A little more of the glutamic form is necessary because it doesn't carry as much HCl). It makes intuitive sense to take less with small meals or snacks, but it's hard to set clear guidelines on how to arrive at the proper dose. Individuals may have to experiment with different doses to see which one does the job without causing discomfort.

When HCl supplementation is not feasible, gradually increasing quantities of lemon juice (citric acid) or vinegar (acetic acid) will often relieve some or even all symptoms. This is supported by the common practice in some cultures of treating gastric discomfort with lemon juice or vinegar. Unfortunately, even though symptoms may be improved, actual nutrient digestion and assimilation are not improved nearly as much as with HCl replacement.

The doses of HCl recommended here may seem high, especially when compared with the usual label recommendations. However, a normally functioning stomach is quite capable of producing much more. Then why not give even higher doses? The fact is that clinical experience shows that these doses work quite well.

Side Effects?

Side effects from HCl replacement are generally mild, taking the form of some kind of GI distress, like pain, burning, gas, or other feelings of discomfort. For most people, reducing or temporarily eliminating the dose relieves these symptoms. Paradoxically, adverse symptoms are most likely to occur in individuals with the lowest levels of stomach acid. This is because these people are most likely to have atrophic gastritis (a thinned-out stomach lining), which makes them much more sensitive to even small quantities of HCl than a normal, thicker stomach lining.

Is It Working?

To monitor the effectiveness of the HCl/pepsin replacement (as well as digestive enzyme replacement), I request repeated follow-up stool specimens to analyze how well protein and other dietary components are being digested. I also look for improvements in mineral absorption, reflected in hair and blood tests. With many individuals, "before and after" blood tests for amino acids give strong indications of effectiveness. Most importantly, we monitor for both short- and long-term symptom improvement.

Pancreatic Enzymes

When the acidified food slurry known as chyme reaches the upper end of the small intestine (duodenum), the low pH triggers the release of the hormone *secretin*. Secretin, in turn, stimulates the pancreas to release *bicarbonate*, which elevates the pH of the stomach content. Also released are a group of *enzymes* to digest fats, carbohydrates, and any remaining undigested proteins. As we have pointed out earlier, if gastric acid secretion is deficient, the pH of chyme may not be low enough to trigger secretin release. Consequently, the subsequent release of pancreatic enzymes may not occur efficiently. A weakened pancreas, a frequent occurrence with aging, can also lead to an enzyme deficiency. (Researchers have found, and I have observed repeatedly, that individuals with diabetes often have inadequate digestive enzymes, too.)

Indigestion or flatulence beginning an hour or more after meals— about the time that chyme would be reaching the duodenum—is often a sign that pancreatic enzyme secretion is not what it should be. Floating stools are a relatively reliable sign that fats are not being digested properly due to low levels of pancreatic enzymes (fat floats on water). Other signs include greasy, smelly stools; dry flaky skin; small, hard bumps on the back of the arm; and impaired dark adaptation ("night blindness"). All these signs are frequently related to undigested foods and resulting nutritional deficiencies.

If pancreatic enzyme secretion isn't stimulated due to low gastric acid secretion, HCl supplementation may be all that is required to remedy the problem.[9, 10] However, in most cases, enzyme supplements do the job better. The most common replacement is an extract of pancreatic tissue, known as *pancreatin*, that is taken from pigs, cows, or sheep. Alternatively, enzymes derived from plants can be used, although they're less similar to normal human enzymes than the animal forms. These include *bromelain* (from pineapple), *papain* (from papaya), and others. Whether the plant-derived enzymes are equal in efficacy to animal-derived pancreatin has not been adequately studied, so I usually recommend the animal forms (except for vegetarians).

In order to more closely simulate the natural process, it is best to take pancreatic enzymes at the *end* of a meal. (I *know* that the bottle labels usually state the opposite. I don't agree!) Taking digestive enzymes *after meals* gives the food adequate time to undergo the "acid phase" of digestion, as happens with normal digestive function. I usually recommend a trial of two to four capsules of pancreatin, bromelain, or papain after meals. If this helps to improve digestion, then I recommend continuing to take them.

Keep in mind that pancreatic enzyme deficiencies usually occur along-side hypochlorhydria or achlorhydria. Thus, if HCl replacement is indicated, pancreatic enzyme replacement probably is also.

Digestive enzyme supplements are generally safe. The most important potential hazard is an allergic reaction, which usually takes the form of loose stools or diarrhea, although a skin rash or other allergic symptoms are possible but rare.

Herbs, Bitter and Otherwise

A wide variety of herbal remedies can produce important beneficial effects on GI function. Many of these are "bitter herbs," which have long held an important place in many different medical traditions, because they stimulate digestion. As the name suggests, when placed on the tongue, bitter herbs, or "bitters," taste bitter.

Studies over the years have confirmed that bitters probably work by increasing the flow of a variety of digestive juices, including HCl, bile, pepsin, gastrin, and pancreatic enzymes.[11-15] It almost goes without saying that bitters increase the secretion of saliva. They may also help head off reflux by increasing the tone of the LES. It is unclear whether we even need to swallow a bit of bitters to obtain its benefits. Some research suggests that it may only be necessary to taste them.[16]

It is thought that bitters may have a "priming" effect on digestion in the mouth, esophagus, and stomach. We may have evolved this response as a means of protecting ourselves from poisons, since poisonous substances often have a bitter taste. Those poisons that don't get spit out immediately might get deactivated by acid and enzymes in the stomach. However they work, though, modern studies confirm the usefulness of bitter herbs like gentian root and wormwood (artemisia) in stimulating the secretion of gastric acid, bile, and pancreatic enzymes.[17-18]

Not surprisingly, it's hard to find good published scientific research evaluating the therapeutic use of unpatentable/unprofitable bitters. One *uncontrolled* study was recently conducted in Germany, where herbal medicine is taken far more seriously. The researchers evaluated the effect of gentian root capsules in 205 people with loss of appetite, heartburn, constipation, flatulence, abdominal pain, nausea, and dyspepsia. They reported a rapid return of appetite and dramatic relief of their GI symptoms.[19]

Among the most commonly used bitter herbs in Western medicine are:

- Barberry bark *(Berberis vulgaris)*

- Caraway *(Carum carvi)*

- Dandelion *(Taraxacum officinale)*

- Fennel *(Foeniculum vulgare)*

- Gentian root *(Gentiana lutea)*

- Ginger *(Zingiber officinale)*

- Globe artichoke *(Cynara scolymus)*

- Goldenseal root *(Hydrastis canadensis)*

- Hops flowers *(Humulus lupulus)*

- Milk thistle *(Silybum marianum)*

- Peppermint *(Mentha piperita)*

- Wormwood *(Artemisia absinthium L.)*

- Yellow dock *(Rumex crispus)*

Bitters are normally taken in very small doses, just enough to evoke a strong taste of bitterness. Bitters are almost always available in natural food stores in liquid form. Sometimes they're derived from just one or two of the herbals above; often they're combinations of several.

For best results, the recommended dose (which varies according to the concentration of the particular product) is "taken straight" or dissolved in as little water as possible to maintain the bitter taste. (That's the point!) Bitters should be sipped before meals. Most studies have shown that, in order to stimulate stomach acid as well as digestive processes in general, it is best to *taste* the bitterness.

Bitters generally work best in mild to moderate cases of heartburn/indigestion/bloating, since in these cases it's more likely that there's some still-functional stomach lining available to be stimulated. Because bitters work primarily by stimulating the secretion of gastric juices, they may have no effect if the stomach lining is severely atrophied.

Even in severe cases of heartburn/GERD, bitters *might* be helpful, but it's best to consult a physician skilled and knowledgeable in both herbal and nutritional medicine before using them, since, in cases of LES malfunction, even a little more acid can aggravate symptoms.

Since I'm less expert in herbal medicine than my colleague Kerry Bone, I refer readers interested in learning more about bitters to his writings on this topic, including his number-one-in-its-field textbook, *Principles and Practice of Phytotherapy* (written with Simon Mills) and various articles (see *"How to Take Bitters"*).

Vitamin B$_{12}$

In cases of achlorhydria, it is an established fact that vitamin B$_{12}$ is neither well digested nor well absorbed. When stomach function is normal, vita-

---

How to Take Bitters
By Kerry Bone, MCPP, FNHAA, FNIMH

The main bitter herbs used in Western herbal medicine are gentian and wormwood. For a reflex effect, bitters do not usually have to be given in high doses. Enough to promote a strong taste of bitterness is usually sufficient. This is typically 5 to 10 drops of the 1:5 tinctures of the above herbs in about 20 mL of water. (Bitters are one exception where drop doses are appropriate.) Since bitters have a priming effect on upper digestive function and work by a visceral reflex (which is slow) they are best taken about 15 minutes before meals. Also, bitters work best if they are sipped slowly, to prolong the stimulation of the reflex. This can be difficult for some people, but will give optimum results.

For a direct effect on the gastric mucosa, higher doses need to be used. About 300 to 600 mg of gentian root before meals would be an appropriate dose. Be careful of such high doses of gentian taken in liquid form, since they can cause nausea in some people.

One question which has vexed herbalists is whether the taste of bitters given in liquid form can be masked,* and yet their reflex activity still be preserved. This is probably the case, since the masking agents will change the conscious perception of bitterness, but the bitter taste buds will still be stimulated.

("The Story of Bitters," *Nutrition and Healing* newsletter, December 1998)

---

*For example, with the intense sweetener stevia.—JVW

min B_{12} digestion and absorption are also normal. But for the entire "in-between" group, ranging from seriously low stomach acid to only a slight problem, there's great variability in B_{12} digestion/absorption and even greater controversy about whether supplemental vitamin B_{12} is useful, necessary, or justified. Since testing for vitamin B_{12} status is relatively expensive and not necessarily precise, I take a practical approach.

Whenever testing demonstrates any degree of low stomach acid, I recommend a "trial series" of vitamin B_{12} injections, which can be performed at home. There are many reasons for this approach. Most importantly, it is safe. The only way to "overdose" on vitamin B_{12} is to fill your bathtub and drown in it! It is inexpensive: Usually, vitamin B_{12}, along with needles and syringes, costs less than one dollar per injection (if done at home). In fact, a trial series of twenty to thirty injections is considerably less expensive than a single test for vitamin B_{12}. Lastly, it is almost always obvious to the individual involved whether vitamin B_{12} injections are useful or not.

A "positive" response to vitamin B_{12} manifests as improvement in one or more of the following: energy, sleep pattern, "nervousness," and anxiety. In a negative response, none of these change. If the response is negative, the vitamin B_{12} injections are discontinued after the trial series. If the response is positive, they are continued, with the frequency adjusted to self-perceived need, often once or twice weekly.

In twenty-four years of following this pattern, it has become absolutely clear that there is a sharp difference between hypochlorhydric women and hypochlorhydric men in their responses to vitamin B_{12} injections. Sixty percent to 70 percent of women report that they feel better with them, and continue them for months or even decades. By contrast, only 20 percent to 30 percent of men notice any difference.

Since vitamin B_{12} and folic acid (folate) are so frequently found together in biochemical pathways, we always add a small amount of folic acid to the vitamin B_{12} injections. Also, because absorption of other B-complex vitamins can decline rapidly after age seventy, we also add a B-complex injection to the vitamin B_{12}/folic acid injections in older people. Both folic acid and B-complex injections are quite safe when given intramuscularly (IM).

Other Helpful Herbs and Nutrients

Deglycyrrhizinated Licorice (DGL)

Before the acid-suppressing drugs came along, perhaps the most effective drug for treating peptic ulcer was *carbenoxolone*, which was a synthetic derivative of the ancient healing herb *licorice root*. The value of licorice* for healing peptic ulcers was first documented during the 1940s in the Netherlands. Although quite effective, the use of licorice was limited by serious side effects, primarily fluid retention, high blood pressure, potassium loss, and consequent heart problems. Carbenoxolone also had these same limitations.

The ingredient in licorice that is largely responsible for these unwanted adverse effects is now known to be *glycyrrhizin*, which closely resembles the hormone *cortisone* in its structure and activity. Just as caffeine can be removed from coffee, 97 percent of the glycyrrhizin can also be removed from licorice. What's left, a product called *deglycyrrhizinated licorice (DGL)*, retains the healing properties of licorice but loses its most important side effects. DGL has been shown to be effective in treating gastric and duodenal ulcers, and it works as well in this regard as Tagamet and Zantac, with far fewer side effects (and no acid suppression).[20-22] In animal studies, DGL has even been shown to protect the stomach lining against damage caused by aspirin and other NSAIDs.[23-25]

Although only a small minority of those suffering from heartburn, indigestion, bloating, gas, or GERD actually have peptic or gastric ulcers, evidence suggests that DGL's mechanism of action makes it also very useful for heartburn/indigestion/GERD. The therapeutic effect of licorice (and DGL)—sometimes called "cytoprotective"—appears to derive from its ability to restore the integrity of the gastric and intestinal lining. It does this by enhancing the secretion of protective mucus in the gastric and duodenal linings. Recall that mucus secreted by cells in the GI lining helps form the barrier that protects that lining from contact with HCl and other digestive juices.

Research shows that licorice raises the concentration of compounds called *prostaglandins*, which promote mucus secretion, stabilize cell membranes, and stimulate new cell growth, all leading to the healing of ulcers.[26†] This is the exact opposite effect of drugs like aspirin and the NSAIDs, which suppress "bad" prostaglandins and lead to the formation of ulcers. Thus, DGL may be helpful for people who are experiencing gastric distress because they are taking NSAIDs.

Since DGL became available in the United States in the 1980s, hundreds of individuals suffering from heartburn, indigestion, bloating, gas,

---

*Licorice root should not be confused with licorice-flavored candy, which may or may not contain licorice extract.

†Prostaglandins are further categorized as "anti-inflammatory" (frequently thought of as "good" prostaglandins) and "pro-inflammatory" (frequently thought of as "bad" prostaglandins).

and even GERD have advised me that regular DGL use brings them as much as or more symptom relief than antacids or acid blockers. However, it's *very* important to remember that neither DGL nor any other symptom reliever (with the exception of bitters in some cases) actually helps correct the usual causes of these symptoms, a major one of which is lower-than-adequate stomach acid–pepsin secretion. Only replacement HCL-pepsin (along with other natural measures) can help normalize *both* symptoms and digestive function, restoring the normal flow of nutrients into the body.

For best results, DGL tablets should be thoroughly chewed and then swallowed with as little water as possible, since it helps heal by direct contact with the cells of the gastrointestinal lining. For this reason, DGL is best taken on an empty stomach. I usually recommend thoroughly chewing and swallowing two DGL tablets three to four times daily with no food one hour before or after a meal. It can be used even more often if it's additionally helpful to do so.

Vitamin C

The value of vitamin C for health is well known, and the idea of vitamin C supplementation is now widely accepted (although there's still considerable disagreement on the amounts to be taken). Many people associate vitamin C with such benefits as relief of the common cold and protection against heart disease and certain cancers. Less appreciated is the protective role vitamin C plays in the health of the stomach, where it provides vital protection against gastric cancer. Many studies have confirmed that low levels of vitamin C are associated with a high risk of gastric cancer and that high intake of foods containing vitamin C (as well as vitamin E, beta-carotene, and others) is associated with reduced incidence of gastric cancer.[27–32]

Vitamin C from food is normally secreted (or passively diffuses) directly into the stomach cavity, where it is converted to *ascorbic acid*, also known as *ascorbate*. Thus, normal gastric juice contains both vitamin C and ascorbic acid.[31] Ascorbic acid appears to exert its protective effects here by at least three routes:

- **Inhibiting the formation of N-nitroso compounds.** Ascorbic acid interferes with the chemical conversion of nitrites from food to carcinogenic N-nitroso compounds such as nitrosamines. As we discussed in chapter 5, nitrosamines and related compounds commonly formed in the stomach are thought to be a major cause of stomach cancer. Ascorbic acid interferes with this reaction.[33–35]

- **Retarding the growth of *H. pylori*.** Colonization of *H. pylori* in the stomach makes us vulnerable to chronic gastritis and eventually to gastric cancer. Vitamin C in gastric juice helps retard the growth of this pathogenic bacteria and, in some cases, may be enough to eradicate it altogether.[36-38]

- **Scavenging free radicals.** Reactive oxygen species, better known as oxygen free radicals, are recognized to cause cancer and other destructive changes all over the body by damaging DNA. As an antioxidant, ascorbic acid from vitamin C scavenges the free radicals in the stomach, limiting the harm they can do.[39]

Taking vitamin C

Many individuals with heartburn/indigestion report that the ascorbic acid form of vitamin C is a stomach irritant, but that the various "ascorbate" forms of vitamin C are well-tolerated. These include sodium ascorbate,* calcium/magnesium ascorbate, and multiple-mineral ascorbates. Sodium ascorbate and calcium/magnesium ascorbate are usually available as powders; multiple-mineral ascorbates as tablets. Higher quantities of calcium/magnesium ascorbate and multiple-mineral ascorbates can contribute to "loose bowels," but sodium ascorbate is less likely to do so.

I usually recommend a minimum total of 1 to 3 grams of vitamin C daily, taken two or three times per day with meals. If "loose bowel" is not a problem, it's advisable to take more.

Other Useful Natural Products

We have described only some of the major natural substances that can be used to help prevent or heal upper GI dysfunction. There are many, many more, including:

---

*There is concern that taking in too much sodium can cause high blood pressure in some people. However, researchers who have compared sodium chloride, sodium bicarbonate, and sodium ascorbate have found that only sodium chloride (table salt) raises blood pressure and sometimes causes edema. Sodium bicarbonate and sodium ascorbate do not.

L-glutamine, Vitamin A, and Zinc

L-glutamine, an amino acid, has many functions in our bodies. For example, it serves as the principal energy source for the lining cells of the upper GI tract. If more energy is supplied to these cells, they have a better chance of staying healthy or returning to health if they are damaged. More than two decades ago, electron microscope studies of biopsy specimens showed that *vitamin A* stimulated healthy growth of intestinal lining cells. *Zinc* (which is often marginally deficient in our diets) has been proven to promote tissue healing. For these reasons, for decades I've included these three nutrients in any program that attempts to improve or heal gastrointestinal function, along with the ascorbate form of vitamin C, and now with DGL. Although there's no systematic research on this combination, many have reported that it works even better than DGL alone.

Quantities of DGL and ascorbate recommended are as noted previously. To this are added each day 1000 mg of glutamine, 40,000 IU of vitamin A (not beta-carotene), and 30 mg zinc (from zinc picolinate).

A Special Circumstance

Very occasionally, individuals with heartburn/indigestion/bloating/gas have a test that unequivocally shows very low stomach acid, but they cannot take even a little replacement HCL-pepsin without *stomach* pain (not esophageal reflux pain). This occurs in cases where the stomach lining is so thin (more severe degrees of atrophic gastritis) that it cannot withstand even a little replacement acid. In those cases, use of DGL, ascorbate, L-glutamine, vitamin A, and zinc in the quantities noted above for six to eight weeks usually enables these individuals to cautiously start HCL-pepsin replacement.

Turmeric (Curcumin)

Turmeric is a bright yellow herb used in preparing numerous very tasty dishes, including many curries. It also has a long history in many folk cultures in the Middle and Far East as a treatment for gastrointestinal and other disorders. What little systematic research there is on turmeric has been conducted primarily in Asia and suggests that it acts as a mild irritant that stimulates the secretion of digestive juices, such as saliva and mucus, both of which can help protect the esophagus and stomach against gastric acid. It may also have antioxidant properties[40-43] and improve gall bladder function.[44] A randomized, double-blind, placebo-controlled trial from Thailand found that taking turmeric (two 250 mg capsules four times a day, after meals and at bedtime) significantly improved common symptoms of dyspepsia such as heartburn, gastric pain or discomfort, belching, gas and flatulence.[45] Other research suggests that turmeric treatment can help heal gastric ulcers.[46]

Capsaicin

Capsaicin is the ingredient that makes red peppers "hot." Although it is widely believed that hot peppers cause indigestion, in fact, quite the opposite can be true. Studies have shown that capsaicin protects the gastric mucosal lining from damage caused by aspirin, alcohol, and probably other potentially harmful agents.[47-48] Capsaicin apparently works by activating a built-in "neural emergency system" in the stomach consisting of certain sensory nerves in the stomach lining. This leads to enhanced local blood flow and protective mucus secretion.[49-50] However, since capsaicin can irritate already inflamed tissue, it should *never* be used by individuals with more severe acid reflux (e.g., reflux esophagitis) or GERD except in consultation with a physician who is skilled in nutritional and botanical medicine.

Ginger

Ginger is a traditional herb that has featured prominently in the cooking and medicine of China, India, and other cultures in Asia for thousands of years. The underground root of the *Zingiber officinale* plant, ginger is made into teas, candies, or capsules, and is added to food. As a "medicine," ginger has been used to "cleanse" the body, in part by improving digestion. Specifically, ginger has been used to treat colds, fever, chills, seasickness, menstrual pains, and other disorders. Modern scientific research confirms that ginger can protect the GI tract in much the same way that capsaicin and turmeric do.[51-52] I recommend ginger for its ability to relieve nausea from nearly any cause, especially in cases of nausea due to motion sickness, which is well documented.[53-56] Recent research has also demonstrated that ginger can help prevent atherosclerosis, possibly by inhibiting the oxidation of low-density lipoprotein (LDL, the "bad") cholesterol.[57-58]

Essential Fatty Acids

Essential fatty acids (EFAs) can help heal gastric and duodenal ulcers.[59-64] Since EFAs are one of the most common nutritional deficiencies, I recommend eating fish, *unroasted* nuts and seeds (roasting nuts and seeds removes most of their EFA content), and salad oils. In many cases, an EFA supplement is advisable, especially for those of us who have dry skin. (Dry skin is usually caused by a deficiency in EFAs, not by a deficiency in skin moisturizers.) Since our diets are usually more deficient in omega-3 fatty acids (which are generally anti-inflammatory) than in omega-6 fatty acids (which are generally pro-inflammatory), I advise supplementation with oils containing a majority of omega-3 fatty acids. Flaxseed and walnut oils are the principal single oils containing both omega-3 and omega-6 in a favorable balance. There are also many blended oils available with similar favorable omega-3/omega-6 fatty acid balance. And never forget to take vitamin E whenever taking essential fatty acids.

Chamomile

The herb chamomile has anti-inflammatory properties, which explains its traditional use for helping soothe irritated or inflamed mucous membranes in the digestive tract. Sipping chamomile tea can help relieve heartburn by soothing esophageal inflammation.

Lactase

Lactose intolerance (the inability to digest the milk sugar lactose) is caused by a deficiency in the enzyme *lactase*. It can cause many digestive problems, including gas, cramps, and diarrhea. For many reasons (including, but not limited to, increased risk of cataracts, ovarian cancer, and prostate cancer), it is best to avoid milk and dairy products altogether, and that's what I recommend. However, some lactose-intolerant individuals prefer to consume them anyway. For these individuals, supplements of *lactase* (lactose-digesting enzyme) are available. Research has shown that lactase preparations can reduce pain, bloating, and other symptoms associated with lactose intolerance.[65] Since all lactase products are not equally effective, it may be best to try more than one if necessary.[66]

Probiotics

Supplements containing "friendly" bacteria can be very helpful for promoting healthy digestion, because they favorably alter the intestinal microflora balance, inhibiting the growth of harmful bacteria (including *H. pylori*), boosting immune function, and increasing resistance to infection. Beneficial bugs such as *Lactobacillus acidophilus* and *Bifidobacterium bifidum* secrete enzymes, including lactase, that aid in digestion.[67-71] Stool tests are available to tell us whether the *Lactobacillus* population of the bowels is adequate or not. These can be ordered with the help of any nutritionally oriented physician. If probiotics are found to be needed, ask that physician for a recommendation, since there are so many probiotic products available that a review is not practical here.

Artichoke

Besides making a healthy and delicious food, artichoke is also a plant with important medicinal qualities. In double-blind studies, extracts of artichoke have repeatedly demonstrated benefits to people with indigestion. Artichoke is particularly useful when the problem is lack of bile production by the liver. As a bonus, artichoke can help lower cholesterol levels and protect LDL cholesterol from oxidation, a major factor in the development of atherosclerosis.[72-77] When taking artichoke extract to enhance liver function, it is best to take a supplement that contains 500 to 1000 mg per day of the main active ingredient in artichoke, *cynarin*.

Mastic, the Natural H. pylori Killer

Mastic is a rare and remarkable product that has been a staple of medicine in the Mediterranean and Middle East regions for thousands of years, but is virtually unheard of in Western medicine. Since ancient times, mastic has been valued for its ability to safely relieve a wide range of digestive disorders from bad breath to peptic ulcers. Now known to have broad spectrum antimicrobial properties, it has recently been found to kill various bacteria, including *H. pylori*, the organism responsible for most cases of atrophic gastritis and peptic ulcer.

The only problem with mastic has always been that it is rarer than gold. Mastic resin, which contains the medicinally active ingredients, is produced only by the mastic tree, known as *Pistacia lentiscus* var *chia*, which grows in just one tiny spot on the entire planet, the southern corner of the Greek island of Chios. There must be something magical in the soil of southern Chios, because, when mastic trees that grow here are transplanted to and cultivated in other places with similar climates, they grow well but never produce their therapeutic resin.

In the time of Columbus, mastic was highly valued because it was the best available treatment for all kinds of GI distress, including the deadly disease cholera. This explains the unusual reward offered to Columbus and his crew if they could find a new source of mastic in their explorations of

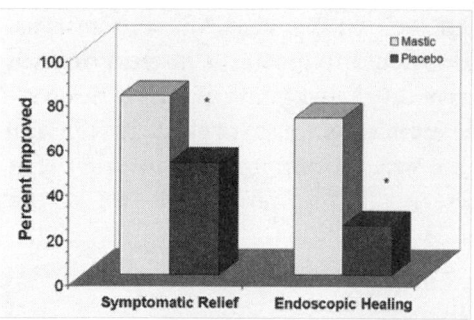

Figure 7-1. Superior symptomatic relief and endoscopically verified healing in duodenal ulcer patients treated with mastic or placebo for two weeks. P < 0.01. Adapted from Al-Habbal et al., 1984.

the New World. In fact, they did find a close relative of *Pistacia lentiscus*, which produced a resin the local natives told them was good for treating stomachaches.

In recent times, the vast majority of mastic from Chios is shipped to locations in the Middle East, where it remains an important therapeutic agent in a variety of GI disorders. Not surprisingly, what little systematic research there is on mastic comes from this area. One double-blind trial from Iraq compared mastic (1 g/day) with placebo in the treatment of thirty-eight patients with duodenal ulcer, which was confirmed by endoscopic examination.[78] After just two weeks of treatment, symptoms improved significantly in 80 percent (sixteen out of twenty) of the mastic-treated patients, compared with 50 percent (nine out of eighteen) of those receiving the placebo. Even more important than symptom relief, though, was the fact that ulcer healing was verified endoscopically in 70 percent of the mastic group, but just 22 percent of the placebo group (aee Figure 7-1).[79] Mastic has also been reported to be effective in healing gastric ulcers in five of six patients within four weeks.[80]

At least part of mastic's therapeutic power probably derives from its antimicrobial properties. Numerous investigators have demonstrated its ability to kill a broad spectrum of bacteria, as well as disease causing yeasts and other fungi.[81–83] Chewing mastic gum for five days has been reported to reduce bacterial dental plaque formation by 41.5 percent in people who were instructed not to brush their teeth during the experimental period. By killing bacteria in the mouth, chewing mastic is also used to help "sweeten" the breath. Due to its malleability, strength, and antibacterial ability, mastic gum has also been used to fill dental carries.

Mastic's ability to kill *H. pylori*, as reported in the *New England Journal of Medicine* in 1998,[84] has finally brought it to the forefront of GI therapies in the United States, as well as provided a mechanism of action for its long-recognized ulcer-healing properties. The report described test-tube research showing that mastic killed several strains of *H. pylori*, including some that were resistant to conventional antibiotics.

In addition to its antimicrobial actions, mastic appears to offer further protection to the GI system from known irritants. This was demonstrated in an experiment in which mastic was found to protect laboratory animals against damage caused by a variety of drugs known to injure the GI tract (aspirin, phenylbutazone, alcohol, and reserpine), as well as by physical stress (cold restraint) and mechanical stress (ligation of the pylorus). The protective mechanism involved here is not yet known.[85] Mastic has no known side effects of any significance.

Mastic is available as capsules, powder, toothpaste, and as mouthwash (mastic oil). Pure mastic resin, direct from the tree (known as "tear drops"), and essential mastic oil are also available.* The resin can be chewed like gum, while the oil can be added to foods. Powdered mastic resin can also be added to foods. For example, in Turkey ice cream is made with mastic powder.

Mastic has been available in the United States for less than two years. So far, the only experience I have had with its use is for those with *H. pylori*–related peptic ulcers. In several cases, 500 mg, three times daily, has been very effective. However, as the last few paragraphs imply, mastic may also be very useful for *H. pylori*–related atrophic gastritis. In such cases, it is theoretically possible that using mastic to eliminate *H. pylori* would allow at least partial regeneration of the stomach lining, perhaps restoring HCL-pepsin production (and overall stomach function) toward normal. However, more research and clinical observation are needed before firm conclusions can be drawn regarding this point.

When to Seek Medical Help; When to Do It Yourself

Before heartburn, indigestion, bloating, and gas progress to more serious acid reflux and GERD, they are almost always treatable by the various all-natural means discussed earlier. It is always best to start out with a combination of dietary changes, drug avoidance, and lifestyle modifications. These will frequently eliminate symptoms and promote healing, particularly in those of us under age forty-five to fifty.

Nearly all of us have had occasional episodes of indigestion from "eating the wrong thing," emotional upset, or "stuffing ourselves" at

---

*Sources of mastic-based products include Life Enhancement Products, Petaluma, California, *www.life-enhancement.com*; Francesco Sirene, Spicer, Peachland, British Columbia, Canada, *www.silk.net/sirene/spices.htm*; Liberty Natural Products, Portland, Oregon, *www.libertynatural.com*; Allergy Research Group/Nutricology.com, 30806 Santana Street, Hayward, California 94544, *www.nutricology.com*.

Thanksgiving. If indigestion is very occasional or the probable cause is obvious, there is no need to be concerned. But if indigestion becomes frequent and persistent, especially if accompanied by heartburn, bloating, and constipation, it is definitely wisest not to ignore it. While only a fraction of those with indigestion will develop more serious acid reflux/GERD with esophageal damage, we don't want this to happen to you! It is always much, much easier to prevent GERD than to treat it.

Step 1: Identify and Eliminate the Cause(s)

Elsewhere in this chapter and book, we have written about many of the known causes of indigestion and heartburn. The first step in a self-help program aimed at eliminating indigestion should always be to identify and eliminate causes, if possible. Most of the common causes are listed in Table 7-1. Remember, causes vary from person to person, and what affects one of us may not affect another. You may need to eliminate only one of these possible causes, a combination of several of them, or even all of them.

Step 2: Bitters to Stimulate the Stomach

If Step 1 isn't helpful, then we should try stimulating our stomachs to work on their own again. *Bitters* are safe, natural stomach stimulants that can restore normal stomach function in many cases. It is always preferable to try bitters before moving on to replacement therapy with HCl and pepsin.

Step 3: Vinegar or Lemon Juice

If indigestion persists, try swallowing one to two tablespoonsful of cider vinegar or lemon juice in as little water as possible during the early part of a meal. If this lessens or eliminates indigestion and/or heartburn, then it is reasonable to conclude that symptoms are a result of insufficient stomach acid.

Step 4: Digestive Enzymes

Sometimes digestive enzymes or "plant enzymes" (e.g., pancreatin, bromelain, papain) taken with meals will relieve indigestion. Taking digestive enzymes is certainly safe, and some physicians advise continuing using them indefinitely to improve digestion and relieve symptoms. *It is very important to understand that symptoms of heartburn/indigestion are usually not due to digestive enzyme deficiency, but instead result from low stomach acid pro-*

duction. As symptom relievers, digestive enzymes are definitely preferable to antacids or acid-blocking drugs. But digestive enzymes do not have the same effect on protein and mineral digestion/assimilation as HCl-pepsin does.

Why is this such an important point? Let's very briefly review the normal digestive process. We chew food, mixing it with enzymes present in saliva. We swallow, dropping the food into the stomach, where it's thoroughly mixed with acid, pepsin, and other stomach secretions. This *"acid phase"* of digestion usually lasts for up to an hour. The food is then propelled from the stomach into the upper small intestine, where its *acidity* stimulates the release of hormones that, in turn, stimulate the release of pancreatic digestive enzymes, bicarbonate, and bile. These mix with food, changing the pH from acid to alkaline. This starts and continues the *"alkaline phase"* of digestion. Both the acid and alkaline phases of digestion are necessary to optimally digest and assimilate nutrients. If we correct symptoms due to lack of *acid* by using *alkaline* enzymes, we may feel better, but we really have not fixed the problem or restored normal digestion.

Step 5: Test Stomach Acid Level

If either cider vinegar/lemon juice or digestive enzymes correct or improve indigestion/heartburn, it is time to consider consulting a physician who can perform a test for hypochlorhydria. We regret to report that, while these tests were once quite common, most physicians (especially "board certified" gastroenterologists) long ago quit testing for stomach acid production. These specialists, who are firm believers in the questionable conventional wisdom that *suppressing* stomach acid secretion is therapeutically necessary and beneficial, uniformly ridicule the idea of HCL-pepsin replacement therapy to make up for a deficiency in stomach function. This attitude is much easier to assume if you refuse even to measure stomach acid secretion. Fortunately, many of these physicians do perform stool tests, which can expose inadequate digestive enzyme secretion. We're sorry to be forced (by facts) to write that very, very few "board-certified" gastroenterologists or internal medicine specialists perform tests to measure levels of stomach acid secretion.

Step 6: Test for Serious Gastric or Esophageal Disease

For more severe heartburn/indigestion, it is frequently best to consult a gastroenterologist first to be checked (usually with a gastroscope) for peptic ulcer, GERD, esophagitis, Barrett's esophagus, or other serious conditions. Once a diagnosis is made, there is usually time to consult a physician who is knowledgeable in using natural treatments before resorting to antacids or (especially) acid-blocking drugs.

What About Self-Treatment with HCL-Pepsin?

For the vast majority of indigestion/heartburn sufferers, a brief "trial" of HCl-pepsin is likely to be harmless and will often bring symptom relief. However, I recommend consulting a physician skilled and knowledgeable in natural and nutritional medicine before embarking on such a "trial."

For readers of *Dr. Wright's Book of Nutritional Therapy* (1979) and *Dr. Wright's Guide to Healing with Nutrition* (1984), this recommendation may seem a bit of a surprise. In both these books, instructions were given for very cautious HCl-pepsin self-trials. However, in the year 2001, there are many, many more of us "just getting into" natural medicine and self-care. A much greater proportion of "newbies" have taken, or are still taking, medication that could adversely interact with HCl and pepsin supplements. The same medications (mostly anti-inflammatories, but other medications, too) can seriously weaken the stomach lining to the point where it cannot handle HCl even if it is really needed. So, if you have indigestion, heartburn, bloating, or gas, and have unsuccessfully tried all the steps noted above, please consider consulting a knowledgeable physician for guidance.

Should Antacid Products *Ever* Be Used?

We have strongly advocated *treating the cause of indigestion* and heartburn (which is very likely to be low stomach acid, variably associated with other factors) *rather than treating the symptoms*. As we've written many times, even though antacids and acid-blockers may relieve symptoms, they are the *exact opposite* of what is really needed both to treat symptoms and to restore normal function.

We have presented alternatives that, used singly or in combination, can relieve symptoms without eliminating the very important "acid phase" of digestion. These should always be tried first, in preference to alkaline-inducing antacids and acid blockers. But what if that is not possible or does not work? To use an extreme example, what if we are stuck on a desert island suffering indigestion and heartburn (too many coconuts?), with no available remedies except for an unlimited supply of acid blockers and antacids? What to do?

Throw the acid blockers into the ocean and rely instead on the antacids until rescuers arrive!* The reason? Antacids neutralize acid and raise the pH, but that is all they do. If we avoid aluminum-containing antacids, and rely instead on those in which the mineral content is mostly calcium and/or magnesium, we are only briefly interfering with the normal digestive process and probably doing no further harm. That is not at all the case with acid blockers, which are much more complex molecules, designed to throw molecular "monkey wrenches" into our bodies' enzymatic machinery. While these drugs indeed achieve the particular effect desired by their drug company creators, they also have a variety of unwanted, and usually unanticipated, effects. If antacids or acid blockers are the only alternatives, antacids are definitely preferable.

Weaning Yourself off
Antacids and Acid Blockers

If you're presently taking antacids or acid blockers, I recommend switching to natural, less harmful methods of dealing with indigestion and heartburn. Since there is no "withdrawal" from acid blockers or antacids, it is safe to just stop them and switch to natural alternatives, as long as symptoms are controlled. In cases of mild-to-moderate indigestion or heartburn, there's usually no problem with switching. In more serious cases, particularly if there's severe acid reflux with ongoing esophageal damage, it's wisest to withdraw from acid blockers or antacids *only* in consultation with a knowledgeable physician.

Finding a Physician Who Will
Treat Indigestion Naturally

It is unfortunate that in today's medical climate, which is dominated by the pharmaceutical and managed care industries, it has become routine for physicians to reach for their prescription pad at the first sign of heartburn and write the name of the most potent acid suppressor they know. Because a significant portion of their knowledge base derives from patent medicine sales reps, medical journals supported by patent medicine company advertising, or patent medicine company sponsored conventions, the average "conventional" medical doctor in the United States knows virtually noth-

---

*In this example, we are temporarily ignoring the adverse effects of acid blockers on fish and all other oceanic life forms.

ing about the natural treatment of digestive disorders. To many of these doctors, natural treatments sound like the latest food fad: "HCl to *prevent* acid indigestion? Give me a break!" Moreover, those "conventional" medical doctors who may be a little more open-minded, are all too often intimidated by their state medical boards, medical societies, or other peer groups, all of whom still disapprove of "natural remedies."

Fortunately, like the rest of us, increasing numbers of medical doctors are beginning to see through the smoke and mirrors offered up by the government/patent medicine company complex. Many of these doctors have taken it upon themselves to learn about natural treatments for indigestion and to recommend these to their patients in preference to expensive, patented, and potentially dangerous pharmaceutical products.

The quickest and most efficient way to find a knowledgeable, open-minded doctor is to locate one who is a member of the American College for Advancement in Medicine (ACAM). All members of this professional organization are skilled and knowledgeable in the prescription and use of various nutritional, herbal, and botanical products. ACAM members have studied and listened to discussions by dozens of experts (even including myself [JVW] on occasion) concerning the biochemistry, effects, and uses of these substances. For a referral to an ACAM doctor near you, contact ACAM at:

American College for Advancement in Medecine
Telephone: 1(800) 532-3688
Address: 23121 Verdugo Drive/Suite 204, Laguna Hills, CA 92653
Internet: http://www.acam.org

Other Medical Alternatives

Although the AMA would probably like you to believe otherwise, there are qualified medical professionals who have letters other than *M.D.* after their names. Many of these doctors, known as *naturopaths*, along with a few naturally-oriented *osteopaths*, tend to have a far better understanding of normal digestive function and how to help restore it, and they usually have considerably more experience in using natural alternatives than the average "regular" M.D.

Naturopathic Physicians

Naturopathic medicine is based on the belief and observation that the human body possesses enormous power to heal itself when given the correct natural materials and energies.

After earning an undergraduate degree (B.A. or B.S.), including premedical requirements such as chemistry, biochemistry, biology, and physics, naturopathic physicians go on to a four-year, graduate-level, accredited naturopathic school of medicine, where upon graduation, they earn an N.D. degree. N.D.'s are educated in all the same sciences as M.D.s, although with less emphasis on drugs, radiation, and surgery, and much more emphasis on nutrition, botanical remedies, manipulation, homeopathy, acupuncture, psychology, and other holistic and nontoxic therapies. Naturopathic physicians place strong emphasis on disease prevention, lifestyle change, and optimizing wellness.

Before licensure, naturopathic physicians must complete at least fourthousand hours of study in specified subject areas, and then pass a series of rigorous professional board exams.

Although naturopathic physicians can be found in every U.S. state and Canadian province, they're currently licensed by state boards only in Alaska, Arizona, Connecticut, Hawaii, Maine, Montana, New Hampshire, Oregon, Utah, Vermont, and Washington, In the District of Columbia, naturopathic physicians must register to practice. In Canada, naturopaths are licensed in British Columbia, Manitoba, Ontario, and Saskatchewan.

To locate a naturopathic physician, contact the **American Association of Naturopathic Physicians (AANP)** at:

American Association of Naturopathic Physicians
Telephone: (703) 610-9037
Fax: (703) 610-9005
Postal Address: 8201 Greensboro Drive,
Suite 300 McLean, Virginia 22102
Internet: http://www.naturopathic.org/

Osteopathic Physicians

After earning an undergraduate degree (B.A. or B.S.), doctors of osteopathic medicine graduate from a four-year osteopathic medical school with a D.O. degree. Their training and accreditation is similar to that which medical doctors receive. Most osteopaths are primary care physicians, but many specialize in such areas as internal medicine, surgery, pediatrics, radiology, or pathology. Residencies in these areas typically require an additional two to six years of training beyond medical school.

Although many D.O.'s are members of the AMA, generally they differ from M.D.'s in their emphasis on the "whole person" and a preventive approach to the practice of medicine. Rather than treating specific symptoms, as many conventional "allopathic" M.D.'s usually do, a D.O. is trained to focus on the body's various systems—particularly the musculoskeletal system—and how they interact with each other. Although D.O.'s can and do prescribe conventional drugs, they are more likely to be open to and knowledgeable about natural remedies.

Osteopaths are licensed in all U.S. states and Canadian provinces to practice medicine and prescribe drugs. To find an osteopath, a good starting point is the American Osteopathic Association (AOA) or the Canadian Osteopathic Association. However, it's always wisest to ask any osteopath's office whether the physician uses natural therapies, as the majority still do not.

American Osteopathic Association
Telephone: (800) 621-1773
Fax: (312) 202-8200
Postal Address: 142 E. Ontario Street, Chicago, IL 60611-2864
Internet: http://www.am-osteo-assn.org

Canadian Osteopathic Association
Postal Address: 575 Waterloo Street, London, Ontario, N6B 2R2
Telephone: (519) 439-5521

Compounding Pharmacists: Back to the Future

Another excellent source of information and useful therapeutic products is the growing number of compounding pharmacies in the United States. Compounding pharmacists can prepare natural medications and herbs for each patient according to their doctor's prescription in the form best suited to the patient's individual needs. Although they cannot diagnose illnesses, they can offer valuable advice to both physicians and patients.

In the centuries before the patent medicine industry took over the manufacturing of nearly all drugs, all pharmacists were compounding pharmacists. As recently as the early 1940s, most drugs and natural compounds were prepared this way. By the 1990s, most pharmacists had been relegated to the role of pill counters.

As everyone knows, the current system basically works like this: the doctor writes a prescription for a standardized commercial drug like Prilosec and either calls the pharmacist or gives the prescription to the patient, who then hands it to the pharmacist at the local drug store. The pharmacist, who keeps a supply of Prilosec pills on hand, reads the prescription, grabs a box off the shelf, sticks a label with the patient's name and dosing instructions on it, fills it with pills, and hands the box to the patient. In many cases a vending machine could do the job just as well (some "advanced" pharmacies actually have machines that do this with popular drugs.)

Fortunately, compounding pharmacies have been undergoing a rebirth, caused by rapidly growing public demand for more natural and more individualized health care, and by economic necessity for the traditional, small personal-service pharmacy. Consumers are increasingly dissatisfied with "nothing but drugs" and are seeking out natural remedies in ever-increasing numbers. Many drug-prescribing doctors are increasingly frustrated with the limited selection of "approved" drug preparations and are working with compounding pharmacists in growing numbers to develop unique preparations and "delivery systems." Many small, traditional, personal-service pharmacies were literally being driven out of business by cost-cutting insurance companies, managed care organizations, and HMOs that sign contracts with giant drugstore chains to provide massive quantities of deeply discounted drugs, or even opening their own mail-in drug outlets. With rapidly increasing consumer demand, the path to economic survival for smaller personal-service pharmacies became obvious: a return to traditional pharmaceutical compounding.

Today's compounding pharmacists can produce literally "whatever the doctor orders," usually in a variety of forms that best suits the individual patient's needs. The pills, capsules, creams, and other forms produced by a compounding pharmacist are virtually indistinguishable from the mass-produced variety, except that they usually do not come with the chemical colorings and shapes the pharmaceutical industry uses to distinguish its products from the competition and discourage "counterfeiting." As an added "bonus," a compounding pharmacist can leave out all unnecessary chemical flavors, preservatives, and adhesives (in patch products), as well as coloring chemicals, and can individualize "bases" according to a patient's allergies and sensitivities.

The quality of individually prepared natural hormones or drugs produced by a compounding pharmacist is generally excellent for several reasons:

- Compounding pharmacists are often more extensively educated than pharmacists who are just "pill-counters." They've taken special training in modern compounding methods.

- They have that extra motivation borne of having to satisfy each individual customer for their individualized prescription. A primary motivation for many noncompounding pharmacists is keeping a "third-party payer" happy. "Happiness" for third-party payers *always* means the lowest price possible, with "patient satisfaction" a very secondary consideration.

- Every compounding pharmacy is licensed and inspected by its State Pharmacy Board, just like all other pharmacies.

- Materials used by compounding pharmacies are the same quality used by the major pharmaceutical companies. All materials used are subject to FDA inspection and the agency's Good Manufacturing Procedures code.

It's no surprise that the FDA and the pharmaceutical industry would like to see competition from compounding pharmacists eliminated, and they have made significant efforts to squash this valuable health resource. So far, this repression has been stalled in Congress and the courts, thanks to the vigorous efforts of representatives of the compounding pharmacists, knowledgeable medical professionals and consumers, and others concerned with preserving one of the last outposts of health care freedom in the USA.

How to Locate a Compounding Pharmacist

Compounding pharmacies are located all over the country, and finding one nearby is not difficult. If there is no compounding pharmacy nearby, nearly all transactions can be carried out via mail, phone, and/or fax.

The easiest way to locate a compounding pharmacist is to contact either the Professional Compounding Centers of America, Inc. (PCCA) or the International Academy of Compounding Pharmacists (IACP).

PCCA provides compounding pharmacists with support in the form of training, equipment, chemicals, and technical consultation on difficult compounding problems. At present, more than nineteen-thousand compounding pharmacists in the United States, Canada, Australia, and New Zealand are members of PCCA. For information about PCCA, including a listing of compounding pharmacists, you can contact them at:

Professional Compounding Centers of America
Telephone: (800) 331-2498
Fax: (800) 874-5760
Postal address: 9901 South Wilcrest Drive, Houston, TX 77099
Internet: http://www.pccarx.com/

The IACP can be contacted at:

International Academy of Compounding Pharmacists
Telephone: (800) 927-4227
Fax: (281) 495-0602
Postal Address: PO Box 1365, Sugar Land, TX 77487
Internet: http://www.iacprx.org/

Is Depression the Result of an Amino Acid and Neurotransmitter Deficiency?

Depression is never caused by a deficiency of drugs! After working with individuals suffering from depression, I am convinced that a considerable proportion of "clinical depression" is caused simply by a deficiency of neurotransmitters, which are (mostly) made from amino acids. (Neurotransmitters are the molecules that "carry the messages" from one neuron [nerve cell] to the next.)

If an individual's history includes a "favorable response" to an antidepressant medication, we can be quite confident that a combination of nutritional therapies centering on essential amino acids will eliminate the depression even better than the patent medication did, and with virtually no side effects. Even if the patentable antidepressant drug is currently being taken, the use of an individualized combination of essential amino acids and other nutritional therapies will almost always allow a gradual "tapering off" of the patent medication without recurrence of the depression.

For depressed individuals who've not taken patent medications, this same treatment is likely to be just as effective in a high percentage of cases.

How can this be? Doesn't it take millions and "kazillions" of dollars, hundreds to thousands of researchers, and decades to develop effective treatments for major individual (and "public-health") problems such as depression? That's certainly true if we're focusing on patentable medications, but if we focus instead on the biochemistry of our bodies (in this case our brains and nervous systems), and work with what happens naturally ("follow the original blueprints"), it's really not that hard to do or understand.

Freud and Electroshock

For most of the first two-thirds of the twentieth century, medical students (your author included) were taught that the mental condition called depression is a problem of psychological origin. In most medical school psychiatry departments from the 1920s through the 1950s, Sigmund Freud reigned supreme. All medical students were taught Freud's theories of "ego, superego, and id," "oral, anal, and sexual," the "Oedipus complex," and so on. Depressed individuals were subjected to psychoanalysis, in which they were instructed in how to (for example) blame their "controlling" mothers and "distant" fathers for their present depressed state.

For "major" depressions beyond the reach of Freud and psychoanalysis, "electroshock" therapy (ECT, electroconvulsive therapy) was sometimes used. As depression had not (and to this day has not) been shown to be due to a lack of convulsion-causing high-voltage electricity in the brain, ECT was not terribly rational or helpful but was used anyway for lack of anything better to do.

Patent Medications

Within a remarkably short time after the marketing of the first "modern generation" of patented antidepressant medications, Sigmund Freud's explanations for depression underwent an abrupt decline in popularity; ECT faded into well-deserved obscurity. It suddenly became fashionable (yes, there are as many "fashions" in medicine as in any other field of endeavor) to describe depression as a "biochemical illness." (If not, how could anyone justify the use of patent medications—chemicals—to "correct" a "psychological" problem?)

Monoamine Oxidase Inhibitors

One of the first categories of patented chemical antidepressants were monoamine oxidase (MAO) inhibitors. A principal effect of these chemicals is to inhibit the enzyme after which they're named, *monoamine oxidase*. Since MAO is active in the normal breakdown of certain neurotransmitters (including dopamine, norepinephrine, epinephrine, tyramine, tryptamine, and 5-hydroxytryptamine, also known as serotonin), inhibition of MAO results in higher levels of all these neurotransmitters. If these neurotransmitters aren't broken down as much as usual, they will, of course, accumulate at higher levels and stay at these higher levels as long as the MAO inhibitor drug is taken. Depression was apparently improved by raising levels of these neurotransmitters with MAO inhibitors. But as patentable molecules never before found present in human bodies, MAO inhibitors had a long and lamentable list of unwanted side effects.

Tricyclic Andidepressants

The next major category of patented antidepressant chemicals to appear was the *tricyclics* (named because of the three-ring-shape of their molecules). The mechanism (or mechanisms) of action of the various tricyclics wasn't as clear, but one major textbook of the time noted that these drugs blocked the "reuptake" of the neurotransmitter norepinephrine by nerve cells (paralleling the action of the "SSRI" drugs noted later). While blocking neurotransmitter reuptake doesn't increase the level of that neurotransmitter, it does allow it do its job for longer than it ordinarily would.

Neurotransmitters and Their Cycles

Let's digress for a brief description of neurotransmitter production and the normal "neurotransmitter reuse cycle." The very large majority of neurotransmitters are made by nerve cells (neurons) from amino acid starting materials ("precursors"). For example, the essential amino acid *phenylala-*

nine and the nonessential amino acid *tyrosine* are processed by neurons to make *dopamine*, *epinephrine* (also called *adrenaline*), and *norepinephrine* (*noradrenaline*). The essential amino acid tryptophan is a precursor of the amino acid *5-hydroxytryptophan* (*5-HTP*) and the neurotransmitter *serotonin*. The nonessential amino acid *histidine* is precursor of *histamine* (which is a neurotransmitter as well as a participant in allergic reactions). One major exception to the "neurotransmitters are made from amino acids" rule is *acetylcholine*, which is made in neurons from *choline*, a naturally occurring metabolite of *lecithin*.

Once produced, neurotransmitters are stored in the neurons that made them until they're used. "Use" consists of release into the space (the *synapse*) between the "producing" or "stimulating" neuron and an adjacent "receiving" neuron. (All neurons can be "stimulating" or "receiving" or both, depending on the circumstances.) Released into synapses from the "stimulating" neurons that produced them, neurotransmitters then stimulate the adjacent "receiving" neuron into action. But the neurotransmitters aren't physically transported into the "receiving" neurons. Instead, some molecules stimulate the "receiving" neuron's outer membrane, and then (in one of nature's many, many cycles) the large majority are reabsorbed by the neurons that produced them in the first place, and stored again for the next use. Only a small percentage of secreted neurotransmitter molecules are "broken down" and metabolized away each time they're used.

Remember how MAO inhibitors are thought to act? The enzyme monoamine oxidase "waits" in synapses for the secretion of monoamine neurotransmitters, such as those named earlier, and "breaks down" a small proportion of them so they can neither be reabsorbed into the neurons that made them nor continue to stimulate the "receiving" neurons. Apparently, even though this enzyme breaks down only a small percentage of neurotransmitters each time they're secreted, blocking that small-percentage breakdown is enough to produce a clinical effect.

Selective Serotonin Reuptake Inhibitors

The 1990s rage in antidepressant patent medications has centered on the "selective serotonin reuptake inhibitors" (SSRIs), the prototype of which is Prozac. (We remember all too well a statement from the front page of the *Wall Street Journal*, which stated that there was a "gold mine" [phrase actually used] in drugs that worked by altering serotonin levels in our bodies.) Remember that neurotransmitter cycle? SSRIs work by selectively blocking the reabsorption (reuptake) of the neurotransmitter serotonin into the neurons that produced and secreted it. The effect is to leave the serotonin molecules in the synapse for a greater-than-natural time period, where, of course, they will continue to stimulate the "receiving" neurons for longer than is normal. Since serotonin is generally a "mood-elevating" neurotransmitter, the individual taking the SSRI will likely feel less depressed. Unfortunately, the list of unwanted SSRI side effects is long and serious.

Nature's Alternatives

It appears that both MAO inhibitors and SSRIs (and possibly the tricyclics as well) exert a major proportion of their antidepressant activity by artificially increasing the number of neurotransmitter molecules in the synapses between neurons, and possibly prolonging their length of activity. How does nature do the same thing without the use of patentable molecules?

Very simply: by making more neurotransmitters in the first place, and putting more of them into the synapses. If there are more neurotransmitters made and secreted into the synapses by the "producing" neurons, then the "receiving" neurons will be stimulated better (better because there are more neurotransmitter molecules) and longer (longer because it takes a longer time to reabsorb a greater number of neurotransmitter molecules), and depression will be relieved, or not happen in the first place!

When working with an individual with depression, I prefer to recommend individualized combinations of all eight essential amino acids. (When supplied with all other essential nutrients—vitamins, minerals, essential fatty acids—our bodies can usually take these "eight essentials" and turn them into all the hundreds of other amino acids—and most of the neurotransmitters—that our bodies require.) However, for purposes of preliminary illustration, we'll first consider the use of single essential amino acids, tryptophan and phenylalanine.

Tryptophan is metabolized into serotonin, the previously noted "mood elevating" neurotransmitter. One might immediately suspect that by taking extra quantities of tryptophan, an individual could raise his or her own levels of serotonin and consequently lessen or abolish depression in some cases, especially those cases affected by SSRI drugs. That suspicion would be correct: In the last year tryptophan was available for public purchase, nearly 14 million individuals bought nearly $200 million worth of tryptophan capsules (at approximately $15 per bottle versus over $100 per bottle for some SSRIs), and the "growth curve" for tryptophan sales was climbing exponentially. By raising levels of serotonin following "Nature's way," and without side effects, tryptophan purchasers were making a serious dent in the market for Prozac and other patented SSRIs.

At this point, we'll pause to reflect on the words of one of our highly paid public servants:

> " . . . Pay careful attention to what is happening [with dietary supplements] in the legislative arena . . . there could be created a class of products to compete with approved drugs . . . the establishment of a separate regulatory category for supplements could undercut exclusivity rights enjoyed by holders of approved drug applications."
>
> —David Abrams,
> FDA Deputy Commissioner for Policy,
> D-C-A Tan Sheet 11, July 19, 1993

Clearly, the use of an unpatentable amino acid to (in many cases) relieve depression effectively, inexpensively, and without side effects just isn't "FDA policy," and something had to be done. By inexplicable coincidence, just as the situation was looking grim for the profits of manufacturers of SSRIs, the "tryptophan contamination episode" occurred, and tryptophan was removed from the open market. Permanently.

I do not make light of the "tryptophan contamination episode." Nearly forty people died, hundreds were made seriously ill, and some have still not recovered. But once the cause of the problem was found (at the Mayo Clinic laboratories and elsewhere), tryptophan never returned for public purchase. (Presently, it's available only by prescription through compounding pharmacies at approximately three times the prior price. As no one has become ill or died from prescription tryptophan, one might wonder why an over-the-counter version of this essential amino acid should be dangerous. But that's a topic more than adequately addressed by FDA Deputy Commissioner Abrams, or his successors.)

Back to neurotransmitters: Phenylalanine is converted by neurons into norepinephrine (and epinephrine). Some individuals have found that taking extra quantities of phenylalanine relieves their depression and even "energizes" them. Although individuals with the genetic disease phenylketonuria (PKU) cannot tolerate phenylalanine, in the rest of us (over 99 percent), no serious side effects of phenylalanine ingestion have been reported, and phenylalanine has had (so far) no "contamination episodes." Many individuals use the nonessential amino acid tyrosine for this same purpose: Tyrosine is a metabolite of phenylalanine on the "pathway" to norepinephrine and epinephrine.

Obviously, individual amino acids such as tryptophan, phenylalanine, and tyrosine can be used to safely raise levels of neurotransmitters and relieve depression. Why do I insist on individualized combinations of all eight essential amino acids instead? Put simply, it's because, at the present time, "we" (science) don't know enough about the incredible complexities of brain biochemistry! (For example, how many of us have read or heard about the use of the essential amino acid *threonine* as a treatment for depression? According to Dr. Eric Braverman, when he was working with the famous Dr. Carl Pfeiffer at the Princeton Brain Bio Center, it was found that threonine was helpful for 18 percent of depressed individuals.) But even though "science" doesn't know as much as it needs to about which essential amino acids do what (and how they do what they do) in the brain, *Nature does know.*

So how do I presume to know precisely (or even semiprecisely) exactly what Nature knows to get the job done? How do I presume to know exactly the right amount of each essential amino acid for each depressed individual?

I don't know. I ask, every time. And the answer is different for every individual.

Before this begins to sound just too preposterous for words, I immediately admit that the "asking" is done by very conventional means: a blood test.

As part of the laboratory evaluation of individuals suffering from depression, I request a "fasting plasma essential amino acid" determination. (Testing is done either at Meridian Valley Laboratories, Kent, Washington [253-859-8700; *http://www.meridianvalleylab.com*], for whom I am a consultant, or at MetaMetrix Laboratories, Norcross, Georgia [770-446-5483], with whom I am not affiliated.) Very frequently, the test report shows that two, three, or more—occasionally all eight—essential amino acids are lower than the normal range. Less frequently, one or two of the essential amino acids are higher than the normal range. Using a previously determined "optimum" number for each essential amino acid (an "optimum" derived from testing many nondepressed individuals), a calculation is performed to determine what percentage of each amino acid is likely to help "balance" all essential amino acids at "optimum" for that individual. (Another thing "science" has very little knowledge about is the effects of "relative balance" of one amino acid to another; once again, I am guided by Nature and what's found naturally in nondepressed individuals.) Of course, the calculation yields different results for every depressed individual, as no two have exactly the same blood test results.

Next, I recommend a quantity of the balanced-for-that-individual blend of *all eight* essential amino acids, ranging from a minimum of 5 to a usual maximum of 15 grams daily. (Tryptophan presently must be prescribed separately and added by each individual to his or her own individualized combination, as the companies that supply individualized amino acid combinations cannot legally do so. The "tryptophan problem" can also be handled by working with a compounding pharmacist, but this solution is usually more expensive.)

> **HOW LOW STOMACH ACID MIGHT CAUSE DEPRESSION**
>
> low stomach acid
> ⬇
> reduced absorption of essential amino acids
> ⬇
> neurotransmitter(serotonin, norepinephrine) deficiency
> ⬇
> depression

Five to 15 grams? That's . . . 5,000 to 15,000 mg a day! Isn't that too much?

The previously-termed "RDA" (officially, "recommended daily allowance"; unofficially and irreverently, "recommended deficiency allowance") for "grams of complete protein" ranged from 50 to 60 grams daily, depending on whether or not one lived in India (no kidding!). Remembering that a balanced combination of all eight essential amino acids is equivalent gram-for-gram with "complete protein," it's obvious that 5 to 15 grams is a small fraction of even the RDA, and won't "overdose" anyone, especially if a test shows deficiency before starting. In my experience, 5 grams daily is an absolute minimum, and 10 to 15 grams daily is more likely to be effective, and also more quickly.

Although there's no way at present to measure directly, the overwhelming likelihood is that low levels of one or more essential amino acids result in low levels of one or more neurotransmitters, with resulting varying degrees of depression. It's also overwhelmingly likely that normalizing low levels of essential amino acids contributes greatly to the elevation of levels of the neurotransmitters of which amino acids are precursors (remember, choline to acetylcholine is a major exception), and thus to the disappearance of depression—especially (but not limited to) those depressions "favorably" influenced by patentable medications that also act on neurotransmitters!

How often does this natural "individualized combined essential amino acid" treatment approach to depression work? Although I have no research grant to help compile exact statistics, experience shows that it will help over 50 percent of depressed individuals, which is equal to or better than the numbers generally claimed for antidepressant drugs. All it takes to predict success is the "fasting plasma essential amino acid" test. If no essential amino acids are low, replacing them is not very likely to be helpful; the lower the essential amino acids, the more likely that normalizing them will do the job.

What, No St. John's Wort?

Aided mightily by the media, many have the impression that St. John's Wort is the major "alternative" treatment for depression. Although, there is no doubt that St. John's Wort is often effective, it should actually be one of the *last* natural treatments to try.

A basic principle of nutritional and natural medicine is *always use the relevant essential nutrients first*, before turning to or adding other natural treatments, whether herbal or any other type. The reason is simple: Since every essential nutrient has dozens of purposes in our bodies, if we have a need for an essential nutrient for one purpose we happen to know about, the chances are nearly 100 percent that we have a need for that essential nutrient for other purposes, which we may or may not know about. Just as we should always use zinc and essential fatty acids for the prostate before we add saw palmetto, we should always explore the use of essential amino acids (and other essential nutrients) for depression before turning to or adding St. John's Wort. To be clear: I am *not* opposed to the use of St. John's Wort. I am *in favor,* as long as all essential nutrients are "covered" first.

Why Are the Essential Amino Acids Low?

As we discuss in detail in this book, the usual reason is poor digestion/assimilation, with hypochlorhydria (low stomach acid) most frequently present.

In Summary

For the reasons stated above, I am convinced that in a large percentage of cases, depression is the result of a neurotransmitter deficiency which is most often due to low stomach acid. In over 50 percent of cases, depression is treatable by supplying (relatively) large quantities of the essential amino acids needed by each depressed individual, along with any supporting nutrients or metabolites. Ultimately, correction of depression in these cases can be achieved by compensating for faulty digestion.

APPENDIX 2
Are Our Faces Red?
Acne Rosacea and
Low Stomach Acid

One of David Flanagan's problems was obvious. His entire face was shiny and pinkish red, more pink around the edges and more red and shiny on and around his nose and the central areas of his face. There were a few small nodules scattered at random on his forehead, cheeks, and chin, and an unfortunately larger one on the end of his nose.

"I'm here from Chicago," he said. "And you can see why! I've had this 'rosacea' thing since I was twenty-two or twenty-three, and I'm forty-one now. I've had more tetracycline than I can remember, and it helps when I take it, but it's been helping less and less the last few years. I asked my dermatologist about cortisone ointment or cream, but she said if I kept using it for a chronic skin condition like this, my skin would just thin out. She's tried other antibiotics, but they don't even work as well as the tetracycline. So my face just keeps getting redder and redder, and now I just use the tetracycline when the pimples"—he pointed to his nose—"get particularly bad."

"Like now?"

"Yeah, though I haven't gotten as many bad outbreaks as I've gotten older."

"Any other problems with your health?"

"Not really."

"Any heartburn, gas, indigestion?"

"Yeah, but no more than a lot of other guys my age. Besides, that happens more when I overeat."

"Tired?"

"I don't think so. 'Course I'm not as full of energy as when I was younger."

I asked other questions about possible symptoms; his answers were negative. After his physical exam, we returned to my office.

"So, what vitamins should I take? That's why I'm here from Chicago. My wife says your clinic does a lot with vitamins and minerals and herbs and all, and that's an approach I haven't tried. If I need to stay a few days, that's OK, I'm staying with my brother here in Seattle."

"You'll just need a day or two at most," I said. "You'll need to have your stomach tested . . . "

"My stomach? The rosacea's on my face."

"I know. But your face is reflecting a gastrointestinal problem."

"Heck of a reflection . . . so if rosacea 'reflects a gastrointestinal problem,' how come no one told me that before? Besides, this gas and heartburn thing is minor, and just started. I've had this rosacea thing for years."

"I don't know why no one told you," I said. "I have an article published in 1948 that says 'every dermatologist knows' about stomach malfunction—specifically low or no stomach acid—in cases of rosacea."

"No stomach acid? What's that got to do with my face?"

"What's tetracycline got to do with your face?"

"Kills germs, I guess."

"Where are the germs?"

"In these pimple things."

"How about all the red skin in between the pimples . . . or when you don't even have pimples? The redness of your skin doesn't go away then, does it?"

"Not really, I guess. So where are the germs?"

"Don't know for certain, but I can guess. When you swallow the tetracycline, where does it go?"

"My stomach . . . . "

"And into the intestines after that. Biggest reservoir of bacteria in the whole body, the intestines, especially the colon. And if we don't have strong hydrochloric acid produced by our stomachs, the entire pH—the acid-alkaline balance—of the intestines and colon is shifted more alkaline. When that happens, "unfriendly" germs are more likely to grow."

"And maybe that's why tetracycline works, at least some?"

"That's my guess. It's also probably why several hydrochloric acid and pepsin capsules taken with every meal help control rosacea as well as or better than tetracycline."

"Because the hydrochloric acid changes the pH—the acidity—back towards normal, and the 'unfriendly' germs can't grow as well?"

"Exactly right. And we get even better results when we use *Lactobacillus acidophilus*—those are 'normal' acid-loving bacteria—as well."

"That's certainly a different approach."

"Almost always works, though. Also, we add injections of vitamin B_{12}, which isn't absorbed as well when our stomachs aren't working, or when we have 'bacterial overgrowth' in the intestines. And as long as we're injecting vitamin B_{12}, we put the other B vitamins in there, too, especially vitamin B_2."

Like most people with acne rosacea, Mr. Flanagan had very poor stomach function. After two years of replacement hydrochloric acid-pepsin capsules with meals, *Lactobacillus acidophilus*, and B_{12} with B complex injections, he flew back in from Chicago to visit his brother again, and came by to show us that his skin was almost normal "for the first time in twenty years."

NOTES

Chapter 1

1. Maton P, Burton M. Antacids revisited: A review of their clinical pharmacology and recommended therapeutic use. *Drugs*. 1999, 57: 855–870.
2. Latner A. The top 200 drugs of 1999. *Pharmacy Times*. 2000, 66: 16–33.
3. Vanpee D, Delgrange E, Gillet JB, Donckier J. Ingestion of antacid tablets (Rennie) and acute confusion. *J Emerg Med*. 2000, 19: 169–171.
4. George S, Clark JD. Milk alkali syndrome—an unusual syndrome causing an unusual complication. *Postgrad Med J*. 2000, 76: 422–423.
5. Fiorino AS. Hypercalcemia and alkalosis due to the milk-alkali syndrome: A case report and review. *Yale J Biol Med*. 1996, 69: 517–523.
6. Galbraith RA, Michnovicz JJ. The effects of cimetidine on the oxidative metabolism of estradiol. *N Engl J Med*. 1989, 321: 269–274.
7. Anon. Diarrhea, skin reactions, and headache following omeprazole (Losec, Astra) therapy. *Curr Prob*. 1991; June (31).

8. Ricci RM, Deering KC. Erythema nodosum caused by omeprazole. *Cutis*. 1996, 57: 434.
9. Buckley C. Pityriasis rosea-like eruption in a patient receiving omeprazole. *Br J Dermatol*. 1996, 135: 660–661.
10. Kraus A, Flores-Suarez LF. Acute gout associated with omeprazole. *Lancet*. 1995, 345: 461–462.
11. Lindquist M, Edwards IR. Endocrine adverse effects of omeprazole. *Br Med J*. 1992, 305: 451–452.
12. Prilosec (omeprazole). *Prescribing Information*. 2000: Merck & Co., West Point, PA 19486.

Chapter 2

1. Krentz K, Jablonowski H. In: Hellemans J, Vantrappen G, eds. *Gastrointestinal Tract Disorders in the Elderly*, pp. 62–69. Edinburgh: Churchill Livingstone: 1984.
2. Carey J, Wetherby M. Gastric observations in achlorhydria. *J Dig Dis*. 1941, 8: 401–407.
3. Lovat L. Age related changes in gut physiology and nutritional status. *Gut*. 1996; 38, 306–309.
4. Hale P. Personal communication. AstraMerck, Wayne, PA. 1997.

Chapter 3

1. Diamant N. Physiology of the esophagus. In: Sleisenger M, Fordtran J, eds. Gastrointestinal Disease, 319-330. Philadelphia: W.B. Saunders Co. 1993.
2. Ibid
3. Freston JW, Borch K, Brand SJ, et al. Effects of hypochlorhydria and hypergastrinemia on structure and function of gastrointestinal cells. A review and analysis. *Dig Dis Sci*. 1995, 40: 50S–62S.
4. Saltzman J. Epidemiology and natural history of atrophic gastritis. In: Holt P, Russell R, eds. *Chronic Gastritis and Hypochlorhydria in the Elderly*, 31–48. Boca Raton, FL: CRC Press. 1993.
5. Prilosec (omeprazole). *Prescribing Information*. 2000. Merck & Co., West Point, PA 19486.
6. Jansen JB, Klinkenberg-Knol EC, Meuwissen SG, et al. Effect of long-term treatment with omeprazole on serum gastrin and serum group A and C pepsinogens in patients with reflux esophagitis. *Gastroenterology*. 1990; 99, 621–628.
7. Lanzon-Miller S, Pounder RE, Hamilton MR, et al. Twenty-four-hour intragastric acidity and plasma gastrin concentration before and during

treatment with either ranitidine or omeprazole. *Aliment Pharmacol Ther.* 1987, 1: 239–251.

8. Lanzon-Miller S, Pounder RE, Hamilton MR, et al. Twenty-four-hour intragastric acidity and plasma gastrin concentration in healthy subjects and patients with duodenal or gastric ulcer, or pernicious anaemia. *Aliment Pharmacol Ther.* 1987, 1: 225–237.

9. Solcia E, Rindi G, Havu N, Elm G. Qualitative studies of gastric endocrine cells in patients treated long-term with omeprazole. *Scand J Gastroenterol Suppl.* 1989, 166: 129–137.

10. Lamberts R, Creutzfeldt W, Struber HG, Brunner G, Solcia E. Long-term omeprazole therapy in peptic ulcer disease: gastrin, endocrine cell growth, and gastritis. *Gastroenterology.* 1993, 104: 1356–1370.

11. Creutzfeldt W, Lamberts R. Is hypergastrinaemia dangerous to man? *Scand J Gastroenterol Suppl.* 1991, 180: 179–191.

12. Mertz H. *Helicobacter pylori: Its role in gastritis, achlorhydria, and gastric carcinoma.* In: Holt P, Russell R, eds. Chronic Gastritis and Hypochlorhydria in the Elderly, pp. 69–82. Boca Raton, FL: CRC Press. 1993.

13. Brunner G, Creutzfeldt W, Harke U, Lamberts R. Therapy with omeprazole in patients with peptic ulcerations resistant to extended high-dose ranitidine treatment. *Digestion.* 1988, 39: 80–90.

14. Lamberts R, Creutzfeldt W, Stockmann F, Jacubaschke U, Maas S, Brunner G. Long-term omeprazole treatment in man: effects on gastric endocrine cell populations. *Digestion.* 1988, 39: 126–135.

15. Pounder R, Smith J. Drug-induced changes of plasma gastrin concentration. *Gastroenterol Clin North Am.* 1990, 19: 141–153.

16. Koop H, Naumann-Koch C, Arnold R. Effect of omeprazole on serum gastrin levels: influence of age and sex. *Z Gastroenterol.* 1990, 28: 603–605.

17. Koop H, Klein M, Arnold R. Serum gastrin levels during long-term omeprazole treatment. *Aliment Pharmacol Ther.* 1990, 4: 131–138.

Chapter 4

1. Krasinski SD, Russell RM, Samloff IM, et al. Fundic atrophic gastritis in an elderly population. Effect on hemoglobin and several serum nutritional indicators. *J Am Geriatr Soc.* 1986, 34: 800–806.

2. Ogilvie J. The gastric secretion in anaemia. *Arch Dis Childhood.* 1935, 10: 143–148.

3. Jacobs A, Lawrie JH, Entwistle CC, Campbell H. Gastric acid secretion in chronic iron-deficiency anaemia. *Lancet.* 1966, 2: 190–192.

4. Gordon-Taylor G, Hudson R, Dodds E, Warner J, Whitby L. The remote results of gastrectomy. *Br J Surg.* 1929, 16: 641–667.
5. Kassarjian Z, Russell R. Hypochlorhydria: A factor in nutrition. *Ann Rev Nutr.* 1989, 9: 271–285.
6. Lazlo J. Effect of gastrointestinal conditions on the mineral-binding properties of dietary fibers. In: Dintzis F, Lazlo J, eds. *Mineral Absorption in the Monogastric GI Tract (Advances in Experimental Medicine and Biology, Vol. 249)*. New York: Plenum Press, 1993.
7. Bezwoda W, Charlton R, Bothwell T, Torrance J, Mayet F. The importance of gastric hydrochloric acid in the absorption of nonheme food iron. *J Lab Clin Med.* 1978, 92: 108–116.
8. Jacobs P, T B, Charlton R. Role of hydrochloric acid in iron absorption. *J Appl Physiol.* 1964, 19: 187–188.
9. Champagne E. Possible consequences of reduced gastric acid secretion on mineral bioavailability from high-fiber diets. In: Holt P, Russell R, eds. *Chronic Gastritis and Hypochlorhydria in the Elderly*, pp. 171-186. Boca Raton, FL: CRC Press: 1993.
10. Ekenved G, Halvorsen L, Solvell L. Influence of a liquid antacid on the absorption of different iron salts. *Scand J Haematol Suppl.* 1976, 28: 65–77.
11. O'Neil-Cutting MA, Crosby WH. The effect of antacids on the absorption of simultaneously ingested iron. *JAMA.* 1986;255:1468-1470.
12. Skikne BS, Lynch SR, Cook JD. Role of gastric acid in food iron absorption. *Gastroenterology.* 1981, 81: 1068–1071.
13. Ivanovich P, Fellows H, Rich C. The absorption of calcium carbonate. *Ann Intern Med.* 1967, 66: 917–923.
14. Carroll H. Personal communication.
15. Ibid.
16. Lazlo J. Effect of gastrointestinal conditions on the mineral-binding properties of dietary fibers. In: Dintzis F, Lazlo J, eds. *Mineral Absorption in the Monogastric GI Tract (Advances in Experimental Medicine and Biology, Vol. 249)*. New York: Plenum Press, 1993.
17. Bo-Linn GW, Davis GR, Buddrus DJ, Morawski SG, Santa Ana C, Fordtran JS. An evaluation of the importance of gastric acid secretion in the absorption of dietary calcium. *J Clin Invest.* 1984, 73: 640–647.
18. Wood R, Serfaty-Lacrosniere C. Effects of gastric acidity and atrophic gastritis on calcium and zinc absorption in humans. In: Holt P, Russell R, eds. *Chronic Gastritis and Hypochlorhydria in the Elderly*, pp. 187–204. Boca Raton, FL: CRC Press, 1993.
19. Pedrosa M, Russell R. Folate and vitamin B_{12} absorption in atrophic gastritis. In: Holt P, Russell R, eds. *Chronic Gastritis and*

Hypochlorhydria in the Elderly, pp. 157–169. Boca Raton, FL: CRC Press. 1993.

20. Russell RM, Golner BB, Krasinski SD, Sadowski JA, Suter PM, Braun CL. Effect of antacid and H_2 receptor antagonists on the intestinal absorption of folic acid. *J Lab Clin Med*. 1988, 112: 458–463.

21. Ibid.

22. Pedrosa M, Russell R. Folate and vitamin B_{12} absorption in atrophic gastritis. In: Holt P, Russell R, eds. *Chronic Gastritis and Hypochlorhydria in the Elderly*, pp. 157–169. Boca Raton, FL: CRC Press. 1993.

23. Krasinski SD, Russell RM, Samloff IM, et al. Fundic atrophic gastritis in an elderly population. Effect on hemoglobin and several serum nutritional indicators. *J Am Geriatr Soc*. 1986, 34: 800–806.

24. Steinberg WM, King CE, Toskes PP. Malabsorption of protein-bound cobalamin but not unbound cobalamin during cimetidine administration. *Dig Dis Sci*. 1980; 25: 188–191.

25. Saltzman JR, Kemp JA, Golner BB, Pedrosa MC, Dallal GE, Russell RM. Effect of hypochlorhydria due to omeprazole treatment or atrophic gastritis on protein-bound vitamin B_{12} absorption. *J Am Coll Nutr*. 1994, 13: 584–591.

26. Ibid.

27. Marcuard SP, Albernaz L, Khazanie PG. Omeprazole therapy causes malabsorption of cyanocobalamin (vitamin B_{12}). *Ann Intern Med*. 1994, 120: 211–215.

28. Koop H. Metabolic consequences of long-term inhibition of acid secretion by omeprazole. *Aliment Pharmacol Ther*. 1992; 6: 399–406.

29. King CE, Leibach J, Toskes PP. Clinically significant vitamin B_{12} deficiency secondary to malabsorption of protein-bound vitamin B_{12}. *Dig Dis Sci*. 1979; 24: 397–402.

30. Wood R, Serfaty-Lacrosniere C. Effects of gastric acidity and atrophic gastritis on calcium and zinc absorption in humans. In: Holt P, Russell R, eds. *Chronic Gastritis and Hypochlorhydria in the Elderly*, pp. 187–204. Boca Raton, FL: CRC Press, 1993.

31. Sturniolo GC, Montino MC, Rossetto L, et al. Inhibition of gastric acid secretion reduces zinc absorption in man. *J Am Coll Nutr*. 1991, 10: 372–375.

32. Henderson LM, Brewer GJ, Dressman JB, et al. Effect of intragastric pH on the absorption of oral zinc acetate and zinc oxide in young healthy volunteers. *JPEN J Parenter Enteral Nutr*. 1995, 19: 393–397.

33. Lazlo J. Effect of gastrointestinal conditions on the mineral-binding properties of dietary fibers. In: Dintzis F, Lazlo J, eds. *Mineral*

Absorption in the Monogastric GI Tract (Advances in Experimental Medicine and Biology, Vol. 249). New York: Plenum Press, 1993.

34. Maltby E. The digestion of beef proteins in the human stomach. *J Clin Invest*. 1934, 13: 193–207.

35. Lundh G. Intestinal digestion and absorption after gastrectomy. *Acta Chirug Scand Suppl*. 1958, 231:1–83.

36. Cater REd. The clinical importance of hypochlorhydria (a consequence of chronic Helicobacter infection): Its possible etiological role in mineral and amino acid malabsorption, depression, and other syndromes. *Med Hypotheses*. 1992, 39: 375–383.

37. Soper H. The clinical significance of indicanuria. *Am J Dig Dis Nutr*. 1936, 3: 564–565.

38. Cater REd. The clinical importance of hypochlorhydria (a consequence of chronic Helicobacter infection): Its possible etiological role in mineral and amino acid malabsorption, depression, and other syndromes. *Med Hypotheses*. 1992, 39: 375–383.

39. Benkelfat C, Ellenbogen MA, Dean P, Palmour RM, Young SN. Mood-lowering effect of tryptophan depletion. Enhanced susceptibility in young men at genetic risk for major affective disorders. *Arch Gen Psychiatry*. 1994, 51: 687–697.

40. Ellenbogen MA, Young SN, Dean P, Palmour RM, Benkelfat C. Mood response to acute tryptophan depletion in healthy volunteers: Sex differences and temporal stability. *Neuropsychopharmacology*. 1996, 15: 465–474.

41. Leyton M, Young SN, Benkelfat C. Relapse of depression after rapid depletion of tryptophan [letter; comment]. *Lancet*. 1997; 349:1840-1841.

42. Leyton M, Young SN, Blier P, et al. The effect of tryptophan depletion on mood in medication-free, former patients with major affective disorder. *Neuropsychopharmacology*. 1997, 16:294–297.

43. Leyton M, Young SN, Pihl RO, et al. A comparison of the effects of acute tryptophan depletion and acute phenylalanine/tyrosine depletion in healthy women. *Adv Exp Med Biol*. 1999, 467:67–71.

44. Shansis FM, Busnello JV, Quevedo J, et al. Behavioural effects of acute tryptophan depletion in healthy male volunteers. *J Psychopharmacol*. 2000, 14: 157–163.

45. Steinberg S, Annable L, Young SN, Liyanage N. A placebo-controlled study of the effects of L-tryptophan in patients with premenstrual dysphoria. *Adv Exp Med Biol*. 1999, 467: 85–88.

46. Cater REd. The clinical importance of hypochlorhydria (a consequence of chronic Helicobacter infection): Its possible etiological role in min-

eral and amino acid malabsorption, depression, and other syndromes. *Med Hypotheses*. 1992, 39: 375–383.

47. Champagne E. Effects of pH on mineral-phytate, protein-mineral-phytate, and mineral-fiber interactions. Possible consequences of atrophic gastritis on mineral bioavailability from high-fiber foods. *J Am Coll Nutr.* 1988, 7: 499–508.

48. Champagne E. Possible consequences of reduced gastric acid secretion on mineral bioavailability from high-fiber diets. In: Holt P, Russell R, eds. *Chronic Gastritis and Hypochlorhydria in the Elderly*, pp. 171-186. Boca Raton, FL: CRC Press: 1993.

49. Champagne E. Effects of pH on mineral-phytate, protein-mineral-phytate, and mineral-fiber interactions. Possible consequences of atrophic gastritis on mineral bioavailability from high-fiber foods. *J Am Coll Nutr.* 1988, 7: 499–508.

50. Champagne ET. Low gastric hydrochloric acid secretion and mineral bioavailability. *Adv Exp Med Biol.* 1989, 249: 173–184.

Chapter 5

1. Finegold SM, Attebery HR, Sutter VL. Effect of diet on human fecal flora: Comparison of Japanese and American diets. *Am J Clin Nutr.* 1974, 27: 1456–1469.

2. Howden C, Hunt R. Relationship between gastric secretion and infection. *Gut.* 1987, 28: 96–107.

3. Heatley R., Sobala G. Acid suppression and the gastric flora. *Baillière's Clin Gastroenterol.* 1993, 7: 167–181.

4. Waddell W, Kunz L. Association of salmonella enteritis w/ operations on the stomach. *N Engl J Med.* 1956, 255: 555–559.

5. Gitelson S. Gastrectomy, achlorhydria and cholera. *Isr J Med Sci.* 1971, 7: 663.

6. Nalin DR, Levine RJ, Levine MM, et al. Cholera, non-vibrio cholera, and stomach acid. *Lancet.* 1978, 2: 856–859.

7. Van Loon FP, Clemens JD, Shahrier M, et al. Low gastric acid as a risk factor for cholera transmission: application of a new non-invasive gastric acid field test. *J Clin Epidemiol.* 1990, 43: 1361–1367.

8. Gorbach S. Infectious Diarrhea. In: Sliesinger M, Fordtran J, eds. *Gastrointestinal Disease: Pathophysiology, Diagnosis, Management.* Philadelphia: WB Saunders. 1983.

9. Peura D, Guerrant R. Achlorhydria and enteric bacterial infections. In: Holt P, Russell R, eds. *Chronic Gastritis and Hypochlorhydria in the Elderly*, pp. 127–142. Boca Raton, FL: CRC Press. 1993.

10. Cash RA, Music SI, Libonati JP, Craig JP, Pierce NF, Hornick RB. Response of man to infection with Vibrio cholerae. II. Protection from illness afforded by previous disease and vaccine. *J Infect Dis.* 1974, 130: 325–333.

11. Peura D, Guerrant R. Achlorhydria and enteric bacterial infections. In: Holt P, Russell R, eds. *Chronic Gastritis and Hypochlorhydria in the Elderly,* pp. 127–142. Boca Raton, FL: CRC Press. 1993.

12. Driks MR, Craven DE, Celli BR, et al. Nosocomial pneumonia in intubated patients given sucralfate as compared with antacids or histamine type 2 blockers. The role of gastric colonization. *N Engl J Med.* 1987, 317: 1376–1382.

13. Goldin B, Gorbach S. Bacterial overgrowth in atrophic gastritis. In: Holt P, Russell R, eds. *Chronic Gastritis and Hypochlorhydria in the Elderly,* pp. 143–156. Boca Raton, FL: CRC Press. 1993.

14. Theisen J, Nehra D, Citron D, et al. Suppression of gastric acid secretion in patients with gastroesophageal reflux disease results in gastric bacterial overgrowth and deconjugation of bile acids. *J Gastrointest Surg.* 2000, 4: 50–54.

15. Pereira SP, Gainsborough N, Dowling RH. Drug-induced hypochlorhydria causes high duodenal bacterial counts in the elderly. *Aliment Pharmacol Ther.* 1998, 12: 99–104.

16. Shindo K, Machida M, Fukumura M, Koide K, Yamazaki R. Omeprazole induces altered bile acid metabolism. *Gut.* 1998, 42: 266–271.

17. Hutchinson S, Logan R. The effect of long-term omeprazole on the glucose-hydrogen breath test in elderly patients. *Age Ageing.* 1997, 26: 87–89.

18. Brummer RJ, Stockbrugger RW. Effect of nizatidine 300 mg at night and omeprazole 20 mg in the morning on 24-hour intragastric pH and bacterial overgrowth in patients with acute duodenal ulcer. *Dig Dis Sci.* 1996, 41: 2048–2054.

19. Lewis SJ, Franco S, Young G, O'Keefe SJ. Altered bowel function and duodenal bacterial overgrowth in patients treated with omeprazole. *Aliment Pharmacol Ther.* 1996, 10: 557–561.

20. Thorens J, Froehlich F, Schwizer W, et al. Bacterial overgrowth during treatment with omeprazole compared with cimetidine: A prospective randomised double blind study. *Gut.* 1996, 39: 54–59.

21. Goddard AF, Spiller RC. The effect of omeprazole on gastric juice viscosity, pH and bacterial counts. *Aliment Pharmacol Ther.* 1996, 10: 105–109.

22. Patel TA, Abraham P, Ashar VJ, Bhatia SJ, Anklesaria PS. Gastric bacterial overgrowth accompanies profound acid suppression. *Indian J Gastroenterol.* 1995, 14: 134–136.

23. Gough A, Andrews D, Bacon PA, Emery P. Evidence of omeprazole-induced small bowel bacterial overgrowth in patients with scleroderma. *Br J Rheumatol*. 1995, 34: 976–977.
24. Saltzman JR, Kowdley KV, Pedrosa MC, et al. Bacterial overgrowth without clinical malabsorption in elderly hypochlorhydric subjects. *Gastroenterology*. 1994, 106: 615–623.
25. Fried M, Siegrist H, Frei R, et al. Duodenal bacterial overgrowth during treatment in outpatients with omeprazole. *Gut*. 1994, 35: 23–26.
26. Theisen J, Nehra D, Citron D, et al. Suppression of gastric acid secretion in patients with gastroesophageal reflux disease results in gastric bacterial overgrowth and deconjugation of bile acids. *J Gastrointest Surg*. 2000, 4: 50–54.
27. Prilosec (omeprazole). *Prescribing Information*. 2000, Merck & Co., West Point, PA 19486.
28. Stevens J. It's a jungle in there. *BioScience*. 1996, 46: 1–5.
29. Mertz H. Helicobacter pylori: Its role in gastritis, achlorhydria, and gastric carcinoma. In: *Holt P, Russell R, eds. Chronic Gastritis and Hypochlorhydria in the Elderly*, pp. 69–82. Boca Raton, FL: CRC Press. 1993.
30. NIH Consensus Conference. *Helicobacter pylori* in peptic ulcer disease. NIH Consensus Development Panel on Helicobacter pylori in Peptic Ulcer Disease. *JAMA*. 1994, 272: 65–69.
31. The EUROGAST Study Group. An international association between Helicobacter pylori infection and gastric cancer. *Lancet*. 1993, 341: 1359–1362.
32. Parsonnet J, Friedman GD, Vandersteen DP, et al. *Helicobacter pylori* infection and the risk of gastric carcinoma. *N Engl J Med*. 1991, 325: 1127–1131.
33. Logan RP, Walker MM, Misiewicz JJ, Gummett PA, Karim QN, Baron JH. Changes in the intragastric distribution of *Helicobacter pylori* during treatment with omeprazole. *Gut*. 1995, 36: 12–16.
34. Kuipers EJ, Pena AS, Meuwissen SG. [*Helicobacter pylori* infection as causal factor in the development of carcinoma and lymphoma of the stomach; report WHO consensus conference]. *Ned Tijdschr Geneeskd*. 1995, 139: 709–712.
35. Kuipers EJ, Uyterlinde AM, Pena AS, et al. Long-term sequelae of *Helicobacter pylori* gastritis. *Lancet*. 1995, 345: 1525–1528.
36. Kuipers EJ, Uyterlinde AM, Pena AS, et al. Increase of *Helicobacter pylori*-associated corpus gastritis during acid suppressive therapy: implications for long-term safety. *Am J Gastroenterol*. 1995, 90: 1401–1406.

37. Kuipers EJ, Lee A, Klinkenberg-Knol EC, Meuwissen SG. Review article: The development of atrophic gastritis–*Helicobacter pylori* and the effects of acid suppressive therapy. *Aliment Pharmacol Ther*. 1995, 9: 331–340.

38. Kuipers EJ, Thijs JC, Festen HP. The prevalence of *Helicobacter pylori* in peptic ulcer disease. *Aliment Pharmacol Ther*. 1995, 9: 59–69.

39. Solcia E, Rindi G, Havu N, Elm G. Qualitative studies of gastric endocrine cells in patients treated long-term with omeprazole. *Scand J Gastroenterol Suppl*. 1989, 166: 129–137.

40. Kuipers EJ, Lundell L, Klinkenberg-Knol EC, et al. Atrophic gastritis and *Helicobacter pylori* infection in patients with reflux esophagitis treated with omeprazole or fundoplication. *N Engl J Med*. 1996, 334: 1018–1022.

41. Parsonnet J. *Helicobacter pylori* in the stomach—a paradox unmasked. *N Engl J Med*. 1996, 335: 278–280.

42. Hansson LE, Nyren O, Hsing AW, et al. The risk of stomach cancer in patients with gastric or duodenal ulcer disease. *N Engl J Med*. 1996, 335: 242–249.

43. Prilosec (omeprazole). *Prescribing Information*. 2000, Merck & Co., West Point, PA 19486.

44. 39. Solcia E, Rindi G, Havu N, Elm G. Qualitative studies of gastric endocrine cells in patients treated long-term with omeprazole. *Scand J Gastroenterol Suppl*. 1989, 166: 129–137.

45. Jansen JB, Klinkenberg-Knol EC, Meuwissen SG, et al. Effect of long-term treatment with omeprazole on serum gastrin and serum group A and C pepsinogens in patients with reflux esophagitis. *Gastroenterology*. 1990, 99: 621–628.

46. Lanzon-Miller S, Pounder RE, Hamilton MR, et al. Twenty-four-hour intragastric acidity and plasma gastrin concentration before and during treatment with either ranitidine or omeprazole. *Aliment Pharmacol Ther*. 1987, 1: 239–251.

47. Lanzon-Miller S, Pounder RE, Hamilton MR, et al. Twenty-four-hour intragastric acidity and plasma gastrin concentration in healthy subjects and patients with duodenal or gastric ulcer, or pernicious anaemia. *Aliment Pharmacol Ther*. 1987, 1: 225–237.

48. Prilosec (omeprazole). *Prescribing Information*. 2000, Merck & Co., West Point, PA 19486.

49. Freston JW, Borch K, Brand SJ, et al. Effects of hypochlorhydria and hypergastrinemia on structure and function of gastrointestinal cells. A review and analysis. *Dig Dis Sci*. 1995, 40: 50S–62S.

50. Prilosec (omeprazole). *Prescribing Information*. 2000, Merck & Co., West Point, PA 19486.

51. Lamberts R, Creutzfeldt W, Struber HG, Brunner G, Solcia E. Long-term omeprazole therapy in peptic ulcer disease: Gastrin, endocrine cell growth, and gastritis. *Gastroenterology*. 1993, 104: 1356–1370.

52. Creutzfeldt W, Lamberts R. Is hypergastrinaemia dangerous to man? *Scand J Gastroenterol Suppl*. 1991, 180: 179–191.

53. Mertz H. Helicobacter pylori: Its role in gastritis, achlorhydria, and gastric carcinoma. In: *Holt P, Russell R, eds. Chronic Gastritis and Hypochlorhydria in the Elderly*, pp. 69–82. Boca Raton, FL: CRC Press. 1993.

54. Jansen JB, Klinkenberg-Knol EC, Meuwissen SG, et al. Effect of long-term treatment with omeprazole on serum gastrin and serum group A and C pepsinogens in patients with reflux esophagitis. *Gastroenterology*. 1990, 99: 621–628.

55. Brunner G, Creutzfeldt W, Harke U, Lamberts R. Therapy with omeprazole in patients with peptic ulcerations resistant to extended high-dose ranitidine treatment. *Digestion*. 1988, 39: 80–90.

56. Lamberts R, Creutzfeldt W, Stockmann F, Jacubaschke U, Maas S, Brunner G. Long-term omeprazole treatment in man: effects on gastric endocrine cell populations. *Digestion*. 1988, 39: 126–135.

57. Pounder R, Smith J. Drug-induced changes of plasma gastrin concentration. *Gastroenterol Clin North Am*. 1990, 19: 141–153.

58. Koop H, Naumann-Koch C, Arnold R. Effect of omeprazole on serum gastrin levels: Influence of age and sex. *Z Gastroenterol*. 1990, 28: 603–605.

59. Koop H, Klein M, Arnold R. Serum gastrin levels during long-term omeprazole treatment. *Aliment Pharmacol Ther*. 1990, 4: 131–138.

60. Mertz H. Helicobacter pylori: Its role in gastritis, achlorhydria, and gastric carcinoma. In: *Holt P, Russell R, eds. Chronic Gastritis and Hypochlorhydria in the Elderly*, pp. 69–82. Boca Raton, FL: CRC Press. 1993.

61. Freston JW, Borch K, Brand SJ, et al. Effects of hypochlorhydria and hypergastrinemia on structure and function of gastrointestinal cells. A review and analysis. *Dig Dis Sci*. 1995, 40: 50S–62S.

62. Bloomfield A, Polland W. Anacidity with cancer of the stomach. *Gastric Anacidity: Its Relation to Disease*, pp. 125–136. New York. MacMillan. 1933.

63. Saltzman J. Epidemiology and natural history of atrophic gastritis. In: Holt P, Russell R, eds. *Chronic Gastritis and Hypochlorhydria in the Elderly*, pp. 31–48. Boca Raton, FL: CRC Press. 1993.

64. Svendsen JH, Dahl C, Svendsen LB, Christiansen PM. Gastric cancer risk in achlorhydric patients. A long-term follow-up study. *Scand J Gastroenterol*. 1986, 21: 16–20

65. Heatley R, Sobala G. Acid suppression and the gastric flora. *Baillière's Clin Gastroenterol.* 1993, 7: 167–181.

66. Ibid.

67. Stockbrugger RW, Cotton PB, Eugenides N, Bartholomew BA, Hill MJ, Walters CL. Intragastric nitrites, nitrosamines, and bacterial over-growth during cimetidine treatment. *Gut.* 1982, 23: 1048–1054.

68. Soybel D, Modlin I. Implications of sustained suppression of gastric acid secretion. *Am J Surg.* 1992, 163: 613–622.

69. Hawker PC, Muscroft TJ, Keighley MR. Gastric cancer after cimetidine in patient with two negative pre-treatment biopsies. *Lancet.* 1980, 1: 709–710.

70. Elder JB, Ganguli PC, Gillespie IE. Cimetidine and gastric cancer. *Lancet.* 1979, 1: 1005–1006.

71. Elder JB, Ganguli PC, Gillespie IE. Gastric cancer in patients who have taken cimetidine. *Lancet.* 1979, 2: 245.

72. Colin-Jones DG, Langman MJ, Lawson DH, Vessey MP. Postmarketing surveillance of the safety of cimetidine: 12 month mor-tality report. *Br Med J (Clin Res Ed).* 1983, 286: 1713–1716.

73. Moller H, Nissen A, Mosbech J. Use of cimetidine and other peptic ulcer drugs in Denmark 1977–1990 with analysis of the risk of gastric cancer among cimetidine users. *Gut.* 1992, 33: 1166–1169.

74. Moller H, Lindvig K, Klefter R, Mosbech J, Moller Jensen O. Cancer occurrence in a cohort of patients treated with cimetidine. *Gut.* 1989, 30: 1558–1562.

75. Wormsley KG. Therapeutic achlorhydria and risk of gastric cancer. *Gastroenterol Jpn.* 1989, 24: 585–596.

Chapter 6

1. Bray G. The hypochlorhydria of asthma in childhood. *Quarterly J Med.* 1931, 24: 181–197.

2. Ronmark E, Jonsson E, Lundback B. Remission of asthma in the mid-dle aged and elderly: Report from the Obstructive Lung Disease in Northern Sweden study. *Thorax.* 1999, 54: 611–613.

3. Bacal E, Patterson R, Zeiss CR. Evaluation of severe (anaphylactic) reactions. *Clin Allergy.* 1978, 8: 295–304.

4. Bray G. The hypochlorhydria of asthma in childhood. *Quarterly J Med.* 1931, 24: 181–197.

5. Wetzel N. Growth failure in school children as associated with vitamin B_{12}. *Science.* 1949, 110: 651–653.

6. Simon S. Vitamin B_{12} therapy in asthma and chronic dermatoses. *J Allergy.* 1951, 22: 183–185.

7. Caruselli M. On therapy for asthma with vitamin B_{12}. *JAMA*. 1952, 150: 1731.

8. Crockett J. Cyanocobalamin in asthma. *Acta allergologica*. 1957, XI: 261–268.

9. Ibid.

10. Harding S. Gastroesophageal reflux and asthma: Insight into the association. *J Allergy Clin Immunol*. 1999, 104: 251–259.

11. Ibid.

12. Bruno G, Graf U, Andreozzi P. Gastric asthma: An unrecognized disease with an unsuspected frequency. *J Asthma*. 1999, 36: 315–325.

13. Pack AI. Acid: A nocturnal bronchoconstrictor? *Am Rev Respir Dis*. 1990, 141: 1391–1392.

14. Harding S. Gastroesophageal reflux and asthma: Insight into the association. *J Allergy Clin Immunol*. 1999, 104: 251–259.

15. Pack AI. Acid: A nocturnal bronchoconstrictor? *Am Rev Respir Dis*. 1990, 141: 1391–1392.

16. Ford GA, Oliver PS, Prior JS, Butland RJ, Wilkinson SP. Omeprazole in the treatment of asthmatics with nocturnal symptoms and gastro-oesophageal reflux: A placebo-controlled cross-over study. *Postgrad Med J*. 1994, 70: 350–354.

17. Meier JH, McNally PR, Punja M, et al. Does omeprazole (Prilosec) improve respiratory function in asthmatics with gastroesophageal reflux? A double-blind, placebo-controlled crossover study. *Dig Dis Sci*. 1994, 39: 2127–2133.

18. Teichtahl H, Kronborg IJ, Yeomans ND, Robinson P. Adult asthma and gastro-oesophageal reflux: The effects of omeprazole therapy on asthma. *Aust N Z J Med*. 1996, 26: 671–676.

19. Boeree MJ, Peters FT, Postma DS, Kleibeuker JH. No effects of high-dose omeprazole in patients with severe airway hyperresponsiveness and (a)symptomatic gastro-oesophageal reflux. *Eur Respir J*. 1998, 11: 1070–1074.

20. Field SK, Sutherland LR. Does medical antireflux therapy improve asthma in asthmatics with gastroesophageal reflux? A critical review of the literature. *Chest*. 1998, 114: 275–283.

21. Harding SM, Guzzo MR, Richter JE. 24-h esophageal pH testing in asthmatics: Respiratory symptom correlation with esophageal acid events. *Chest*. 1999, 115: 654–659.

22. Irwin RS, Curley FJ, French CL. Difficult-to-control asthma. Contributing factors and outcome of a systematic management protocol. *Chest*. 1993, 103: 1662–1669.

23. Harding S. Gastroesophageal reflux and asthma: Insight into the association. *J Allergy Clin Immunol*. 1999, 104: 251–259.

24. Bray G. The hypochlorhydria of asthma in childhood. *Quarterly J Med.* 1931, 24: 181–197.

25. Knowles F, Decker H. Gastric acidity and acne vulgaris. *Arch Dermatol Syphilology.* 1926, 13: 215–218.

26. Rawls W, Ancona V. Chronic urticaria associated with hypochlorhydria or achlorhydria. *Rev Gastroenterol.* 1951, 18: 267–271.

27. Tedesco A, Lynch P. Association of dermatitis herpetiformis and pernicious anemia. *Arch Dermatol.* 1979, 115: 1117.

28. Andersson H, Dotevall G, Mobacken H. Gastric secretion of acid and intrinsic factor in dermatitis herpetiformis. *Scand J Gastroenterol.* 1971, 6: 411–416.

29. Gillberg R, Dotevall G, Ahren C. Chronic inflammatory bowel disease in patients with coeliac disease. *Scand J Gastroenterol.* 1982, 17: 491–496.

30. Fravel R. The occurrence of hypochlorhydria in gall-ballder disease. *Am J Med.* 1920, 159: 512–517.

31. Capper WM, Butler TJ, Kilby JO, Gibson MJ. Gallstones, gastric secretion, and flatulent dyspepsia. *Lancet.* 1967, 1: 413–415.

32. Spivacke C, Golob M. Depression of hydrochloric acid secretion in allergic conditons. *Rev Gastroenterol.* 1942, 9: 376–379.

33. Milocco C, Torre G, Ventura A. Gastro-oesophageal reflux and cows' milk protein allergy. *Arch Dis Child.* 1997, 77: 183–184.

34. Schrander JJ, van den Bogart JP, Forget PP, Schrander-Stumpel CT, Kuijten RH, Kester AD. Cow's milk protein intolerance in infants under 1 year of age: A prospective epidemiological study. *Eur J Pediatr.* 1993, 152: 640–644.

35. Schrander JJ, Oudsen S, Forget PP, Kuijten RH. Follow up study of cow's milk protein intolerant infants. *Eur J Pediatr.* 1992, 151: 783–785.

36. Forget P, Arends JW. Cow's milk protein allergy and gastro-oesophageal reflux. *Eur J Pediatr.* 1985, 144: 298–300.

37. Staiano A, Troncone R, Simeone D, et al. Differentiation of cows' milk intolerance and gastro-oesophageal reflux. *Arch Dis Child.* 1995, 73: 439–442.

38. Cavataio F, Carroccio A, Iacono G. Milk-induced reflux in infants less than one year of age. *J Pediatr Gastroenterol Nutr.* 2000, 30: S36–S44.

39. Cavataio F, Iacono G, Montalto G, et al. Gastroesophageal reflux associated with cow's milk allergy in infants: which diagnostic examinations are useful? *Am J Gastroenterol.* 1996, 91: 1215–1220.

40. Iacono G, Carroccio A, Cavataio F, et al. Gastroesophageal reflux and cow's milk allergy in infants: A prospective study. *J Allergy Clin Immunol.* 1996, 97: 822–827.

41. Paronen J, Knip M, Savilahti E, et al. Effect of cow's milk exposure and maternal type 1 diabetes on cellular and humoral immunization to dietary insulin in infants at genetic risk for type 1 diabetes. Finnish Trial to Reduce IDDM in the Genetically at Risk Study Group. *Diabetes*. 2000, 49: 1657–1665.

42. Vaarala O, Knip M, Paronen J, et al. Cow's milk formula feeding induces primary immunization to insulin in infants at genetic risk for type 1 diabetes. *Diabetes*. 1999, 48: 1389–1394.

43. Kokkonen J, Simila S, Herva R. Impaired gastric function in children with cow's milk intolerance. *Eur J Pediatr.* 1979, 132: 1–6.

44. Gardner ML. Gastrointestinal absorption of intact proteins. *Ann Rev Nutr.* 1988, 8: 329–350.

45. Walker WA. Antigen absorption from the small intestine and gastrointestinal disease. *Pediatr Clin North Am.* 1975, 22: 731–746.

46. Walker WA. Gastrointestinal host defence: Importance of gut closure in control of macromolecular transport. *Ciba Found Symp.* 1979, 201–219.

47. Walker WA. Uptake of antigens: Role in gastrointestinal disease. *Acta Paediatr Jpn.* 1994, 36: 597–610.

48. Lichtman SN, Wang J, Sartor RB, et al. Reactivation of arthritis induced by small bowel bacterial overgrowth in rats: Role of cytokines, bacteria, and bacterial polymers. *Infect Immun.* 1995, 63: 2295–2301.

49. Walker WA. Antigen absorption from the small intestine and gastrointestinal disease. *Pediatr Clin North Am.* 1975, 22: 731–746.

50. Miller AL. Therapeutic considerations of L-glutamine: a review of the literature. *Altern Med Rev.* 1999, 4: 239–248.

51. Moneret-Vautrin DA, Kanny G, Guerin L, Flabbee J, Lemerdy P. [The multifood allergy syndrome]. *Allerg Immunol (Paris).* 2000, 32: 12–15.

52. Unno N, Fink MP. Intestinal epithelial hyperpermeability. Mechanisms and relevance to disease. *Gastroenterol Clin North Am.* 1998, 27: 289–307.

53. Kovacs T, Kun L, Schmelczer M, Wagner L, Davin JC, Nagy J. Do intestinal hyperpermeability and the related food antigens play a role in the progression of IgA nephropathy? I. Study of intestinal permeability. *Am J Nephrol.* 1996, 16: 500–505.

54. Reunala T, Collin P. Diseases associated with dermatitis herpetiformis. *Br J Dermatol.* 1997, 136: 315–318.

55. Fries JF. Assessing and understanding patient risk. *Scand J Rheumatol Suppl.* 1992, 92: 21–24.

56. Jones M, Wang H, Peskar B, et al. Inhibition of angiogenesis by non-steroidal anti-inflammatory drugs: Insight into mechanisms and implications for cancer growth and ulcer healing. *Nature Med.* 1999, 5: 1418–1423.

57. Woodwark A, Wallis R. The relation of the gastric secretion to rheumatoid arthritis. *Lancet,* October 5, 1912: 942–945.

58. de Witte TJ, Geerdink PJ, Lamers CB, Boerbooms AM, van der Korst JK. Hypochlorhydria and hypergastrinaemia in rheumatoid arthritis. *Ann Rheum Dis.* 1979, 38: 14–17.

59. Henriksson K, Uvnas-Moberg K, Nord CE, Johansson C, Gullberg R. Gastrin, gastric acid secretion, and gastric microflora in patients with rheumatoid arthritis. *Ann Rheum Dis.* 1986, 45: 475–483.

60. Hartung E, Steinbrocker O. Gastric acidity in chronic arthritis. *Ann Intern Med.* 1935, 9: 252–257.

61. Marcolongo R, Bayeli PF, Montagnani M. Gastrointestinal involvement in rheumatoid arthritis: A biopsy study. *J Rheumatol.* 1979, 6: 163–173.

62. Rowden DR, Taylor IL, Richter JA, Pinals RS, Levine RA. Is hypergastrinaemia associated with rheumatoid arthritis? *Gut.* 1978, 19: 1064–1067.

63. Rooney PJ, Dick WC, Imrie RC, Turner D, Buchanan KD, Ardill J. On the relationship between gastrin, gastric secretion, and adjuvant arthritis in rats. *Ann Rheum Dis.* 1978, 37: 432–435.

64. Edström G. Magensekretion und Grundumsatz bei den chronischen rheumatischen Arthritiden. *Acta Med Scand.* 1939, 99: 228–256.

65. Lucchesi O, Lucchesi M. Gastric acidity and rheumatoid arthritis. *Gastroenterology.* 1945, 5: 299–302.

66. Henriksson K, Uvnas-Moberg K, Nord CE, Johansson C, Gullberg R. Gastrin, gastric acid secretion, and gastric microflora in patients with rheumatoid arthritis. *Ann Rheum Dis.* 1986, 45: 475–483.

67. Marcolongo R, Bayeli PF, Montagnani M. Gastrointestinal involvement in rheumatoid arthritis: A biopsy study. *J Rheumatol.* 1979, 6: 163–173.

68. Olhagen B. Intestinal *Clostridium perfringens* in arthritis and allied conditions. In: Dumonde D, ed. *Infection and Immunology in the Rheumatic Diseases*, pp. 141–145. London: Blackwell Scientific Publications. 1974.

69. NSAID and the leaky gut. *Lancet.* 1985, 1: 218–219.

70. Rooney PJ, Jenkins RT. Nonsteroidal antiinflammatory drugs (NSAID's) and the bowel mucosa: Changes in intestinal permeability may not be due to changes in prostaglandins. *Clin Exp Rheumatol.* 1990, 8: 328–329.

71. Raskin JB. Gastrointestinal effects of nonsteroidal anti-inflammatory therapy. *Am J Med*. 1999, 106: 3S–12S.
72. Fravel R. The occurrence of hypochlorhydria in gall-ballder disease. *Am J Med*. 1920, 159: 512–517.
73. Capper WM, Butler TJ, Kilby JO, Gibson MJ. Gallstones, gastric secretion, and flatulent dyspepsia. *Lancet*. 1967, 1: 413–415.
74. Breneman J. Allergy elimination diet as the most effective gallbladder diet. *Ann Allergy*. 1968, 26: 83–87.
75. Hicklin J, et al. The effect of diet in rheumatoid arthritis. *Clin Allergy*. 1980, 10: 463.
76. Schrander JJ, Oudsen S, Forget PP, Kuijten RH. Follow up study of cow's milk protein intolerant infants. *Eur J Pediatr*. 1992, 151: 783–785.
77. Haugen MA, Kjeldsen-Kragh J, Forre O. A pilot study of the effect of an elemental diet in the management of rheumatoid arthritis. *Clin Exp Rheumatol*. 1994, 12: 275–279.
78. De Vita S, Bombardieri S. [The diet therapy of rheumatic diseases.] *Recenti Prog Med*. 1992, 83: 707–718.
79. van de Laar MA, van der Korst JK. Food intolerance in rheumatoid arthritis. I. A double blind, controlled trial of the clinical effects of elimination of milk allergens and azo dyes. *Ann Rheum Dis*. 1992, 51: 298–302.
80. Wright J, Gaby A. *The Patient's Book of Natural Healing*. Rocklin, CA: Prima Publishing Co. 1999.
81. Anderson J, et al. Hyperreactivity to cow's milk in an infant with LE and tart cell phenomenon. *J Pediatr*. 1974, 84: 59–67.
82. Cooke H, Reading C. Dietary intervention in systemic lupus erythematosus: 4 cases of clinical remission and reversal of abnormal pathology. *Int Clin Nutr Rev*. 1985, 5: 166–176.

Chapter 7

1. Rappaport E. Achlorhydria: Associated symptoms and response to hydrochloric acid. *N Engl J Med*. 1955, 252: 802–805.
2. Cho MK, Shohara R, Schissel A, Rennie D. Policies on faculty conflicts of interest at US universities. *JAMA*. 2000, 284: 2203–2208.
3. Boyd EA, Bero LA. Assessing faculty financial relationships with industry: A case study. *JAMA*. 2000, 284: 2209–2214.
4. Angell M. Is academic medicine for sale? *N Engl J Med*. 2000, 342: 1516–1518.
5. Angell M. The pharmaceutical industry—to whom is it accountable? *N Engl J Med*. 2000, 342: 1902–1904.

6. Dressman JB, Berardi RR, Dermentzoglou LC, et al. Upper gastrointestinal (GI) pH in young, healthy men and women. *Pharm Res*. 1990, 7: 756–761.

7. Andres MR, Jr., Bingham JR. Tubeless gastric analysis with a radiotelemetering pill (Heidelberg capsule). *Can Med Assoc J*. 1970, 102: 1087–1089.

8. Richter J. Gastroesophageal reflux disease. *Curr Pract Med*. 1999, 2: 2307–2315.

9. Suarez F, Leavitt M, Adshead J, Barkin J. Pancreatic supplements reduce symptomatic response of healthy subjects to a high fat meal. *Dig Dis Sci*. 1999, 44: 1317–1321.

10. Valerio D, Whyte EH, Schlamm HT, Ruggiero JA, Blackburn GL. Clinical effectiveness of a pancreatic enzyme supplement. *J Parenter Enteral Nutr*. 1981, 5: 110–114.

11. Wolf S, Mack M. Experimental study of the action of bitters on the stomach of a fistulous human subject. *Drug Standards*. 1956, 24: 98–101.

12. Herman JH, Nolan DS. A bitter cure. *N Engl J Med*. 1981, 305: 1654.

13. Moorehead L. Contributions to the physiology of the stomach. XXVIII. Further studies on the action of the bitter tonic on the secretion of gastric juice. *J Pharmacol Exper Therap*. 1915, 7: 577–589.

14. Ogeto J, Maitai C. The scientific basis for the use of *Strychnos henningsii (GLIG)* plant material to stimulate appetite. *E African Med J*. 1983, 60: 603–607.

15. Carlson A, Torchiani B, Hallock R. Contributions to the physiology of the stomach. XXI. The supposed actions of the bitter tonic on the secretion of gastric juice in man and dog. *JAMA*. 1915, 64: 15–17.

16. Bone K. Bitters—still a valuable concept. *Nutrition & Healing Newsletter*. 1998, 5: 3–7.

17. Baumann I, Glatzel H, Muth H. Untersuchungen der Wirkungen von Wermut (*Artemisia absinthium L.*) auf die Gallenund Pankreassaft-Sekretion des Menschen. *Zeitschrift fur Allgemeinmedizin*. 1975; 17: 784–791.

18. Glatzel H, Hackenberg K. Rontgenologische untersuchungen der Wirkungen von bittermitteln auf die verdauuungsorgane. *Planta Medica*. 1967, 3: 223–232.

19. Wegener T. Anwendung eines Trockenextraktes aus Gentianae luteae radix bei dyspeptischem Symptomkomplex. *Zeitschrift für Phytotherapie*. 1998, 19: 163–164.

20. Glick L. Deglycyrrhizinated liquorice for peptic ulcer. *Lancet*. 1982, 2: 817.

21. Turpie AG, Runcie J, Thomson TJ. Clinical trial of deglyrhizinized liquorice in gastric ulcer. *Gut.* 1969, 10: 299–302.
22. Kassir ZA. Endoscopic controlled trial of four drug regimens in the treatment of chronic duodenal ulceration. *Ir Med J.* 1985, 78: 153–156.
23. Russell RI, Morgan RJ, Nelson LM. Studies on the protective effect of deglycyrrhinised liquorice against aspirin (ASA) and ASA plus bile acid-induced gastric mucosal damage, and ASA absorption in rats. *Scand J Gastroenterol Suppl.* 1984, 92: 97–100.
24. Dehpour AR, Zolfaghari ME, Samadian T, Vahedi Y. The protective effect of liquorice components and their derivatives against gastric ulcer induced by aspirin in rats. *J Pharm Pharmacol.* 1994, 46: 148–149.
25. Dehpour A, Zolfaghari M, Samadian T, et al. Antiulcer activities of liquorice and its derivatives in experimental gastric lesion induced by ubuprofen in rats. *Int J Pharm.* 1995, 119: 133–138.
26. Baker ME. Licorice and enzymes other than 11 beta-hydroxysteroid dehydrogenase: An evolutionary perspective. *Steroids.* 1994, 59: 136–141.
27. Correa P, Malcom G, Schmidt B, et al. Review article: Antioxidant micronutrients and gastric cancer. *Aliment Pharmacol Ther.* 1998, 12 Suppl 1: 73–82.
28. Ekstrom AM, Serafini M, Nyren O, Hansson LE, Ye W, Wolk A. Dietary antioxidant intake and the risk of cardia cancer and noncardia cancer of the intestinal and diffuse types: A population-based case-control study in Sweden. *Int J Cancer.* 2000, 87: 133–140.
29. Zullo A, Rinaldi V, Hassan C, et al. Ascorbic acid and intestinal metaplasia in the stomach: a prospective, randomized study [In Process Citation]. *Aliment Pharmacol Ther.* 2000, 14: 1303–1309.
30. Webb PM, Bates CJ, Palli D, Forman D. Gastric cancer, gastritis and plasma vitamin C: results from an international correlation and cross-sectional study. The Eurogast Study Group. *Int J Cancer.* 1997, 73: 684–689.
31. Sobala GM, Schorah CJ, Sanderson M, et al. Ascorbic acid in the human stomach. *Gastroenterology.* 1989, 97: 357–363.
32. Sobala GM, Schorah CJ, Pignatelli B, et al. High gastric juice ascorbic acid concentrations in members of a gastric cancer family. *Carcinogenesis.* 1993, 14: 291–292.
33. Mirvish SS, Pelfrene AF, Garcia H, Shubik P. Effect of sodium ascorbate on tumor induction in rats treated with morpholine and sodium nitrite, and with nitrosomorpholine. *Cancer Lett.* 1976, 2: 101–108.

34. Mirvish SS. Effects of vitamins C and E on N-nitroso compound formation, carcinogenesis, and cancer. *Cancer.* 1986, 58: 1842–1850.

35. Wagner DA, Shuker DE, Bilmazes C, Obiedzinski M, Young VR, Tannenbaum SR. Modulation of endogenous synthesis of N-nitrosamino acids in humans. *IARC Sci Publ.* 1984, 57: 223–229.

36. Zullo A, Rinaldi V, Hassan C, et al. Ascorbic acid and intestinal metaplasia in the stomach: a prospective, randomized study [In Process Citation]. *Aliment Pharmacol Ther.* 2000, 14: 1303–1309.

37. Jarosz M, Dzieniszewski J, Dabrowska-Ufniarz E, Wartanowicz M, Ziemlanski S, Reed PI. Effects of high dose vitamin C treatment on *Helicobacter pylori* infection and total vitamin C concentration in gastric juice. *Eur J Cancer Prev.* 1998, 7: 449–454.

38. Zhang HM, Wakisaka N, Maeda O, Yamamoto T. Vitamin C inhibits the growth of a bacterial risk factor for gastric carcinoma: *Helicobacter pylori. Cancer.* 1997, 80: 1897–1903.

39. Drake IM, Davies MJ, Mapstone NP, et al. Ascorbic acid may protect against human gastric cancer by scavenging mucosal oxygen radicals. *Carcinogenesis.* 1996, 17: 559–562.

40. Rafatullah S, Tariq M, Al-Yahya M, Mossa J, Ageel A. Evaluation of turmeric (*Curcuma longa*) for gastric and duodenal antiulcer activity. *J Ethnopharmacol.* 1990, 29: 25–34.

41. Selvam R, Subramanian L, Gayathri R, Angayarkanni N. The anti-oxidant activity of turmeric (*Curcuma longa*). *J Ethnopharmacol.* 1995, 47: 59–67.

42. Kositchaiwat C, Kositchaiwat S, Havanondha J. *Curcuma longa* Linn. in the treatment of gastric ulcer, comparison to liquid antacid: a controlled clinical trial. *J Med Assoc Thai.* 1993, 76: 601–605.

43. Thamlikitkul V, Dechatiwongse T, Chantrakul C, et al. Randomized double blind study of *Curcuma domestica* val. for dyspepsia. *J Med Assoc Thai.* 1989, 72: 614–619.

44. Ramprasad C, Dirsi M. Indian Medicinal Plants: Curcuma longa—effect of curcumin and the essential oils of C. longa on bile secretion. *J Sci Ind Research (India).* 1956, 15: 262–265.

45. Thamlikitkul V, Dechatiwongse T, Chantrakul C, et al. Randomized double blind study of *Curcuma domestica* val. for dyspepsia. *J Med Assoc Thai.* 1989, 72: 614–619.

46. Kositchaiwat C, Kositchaiwat S, Havanondha J. *Curcuma longa* Linn. in the treatment of gastric ulcer, comparison to liquid antacid: a controlled clinical trial. *J Med Assoc Thai.* 1993, 76: 601–605.

47. Foschi D, Del Soldato P. Effects of capsaicin on ethanol damage in the rat [letter; comment]. *Gastroenterology.* 1991, 100:1155–1156.

48. Holzer P, Pabst MA, Lippe IT. Intragastric capsaicin protects against aspirin-induced lesion formation and bleeding in the rat gastric mucosa. *Gastroenterology*. 1989, 96: 1425–1433.

49. Holzer P, Pabst MA, Lippe IT, et al. Afferent nerve-mediated protection against deep mucosal damage in the rat stomach [see comments]. *Gastroenterology*. 1990, 98:838–848.

50. Holzer P, Lippe IT. Stimulation of afferent nerve endings by intragastric capsaicin protects against ethanol-induced damage of gastric mucosa. *Neuroscience*. 1988, 27: 981–987.

51. Ahmed RS, Seth V, Pasha ST, Banerjee BD. Influence of dietary ginger (*Zingiber officinales Rosc*) on oxidative stress induced by malathion in rats. *Food Chem Toxicol*. 2000, 38: 443–450.

52. Platel K, Srinivasan K. Influence of dietary spices and their active principles on pancreatic digestive enzymes in albino rats. *Nahrung*. 2000, 44: 42–46.

53. Ernst E, Pittler MH. Efficacy of ginger for nausea and vomiting: a systematic review of randomized clinical trials. *Br J Anaesth*. 2000, 84 : 367–371.

54. Jewell D, Young G. Interventions for nausea and vomiting in early pregnancy. *Cochrane Database Syst Rev*. 2000, 2.

55. Micklefield GH, Redeker Y, Meister V, Jung O, Greving I, May B. Effects of ginger on gastroduodenal motility. *Int J Clin Pharmacol Ther*. 1999, 37: 341–346.

56. Langner E, Greifenberg S, Gruenwald J. Ginger: History and use. *Adv Ther*. 1998, 15: 25–44.

57. Fuhrman B, Rosenblat M, Hayek T, Coleman R, Aviram M. Ginger extract consumption reduces plasma cholesterol, inhibits LDL oxidation and attenuates development of atherosclerosis in atherosclerotic, apolipoprotein E-deficient mice. *J Nutr*. 2000, 130: 1124–1131.

58. Shobana S, Naidu KA. Antioxidant activity of selected Indian spices. *Prostaglandins Leukot Essent Fatty Acids*. 2000, 62: 107–110.

59. al-Shabanah OA. Effect of evening primrose oil on gastric ulceration and secretion induced by various ulcerogenic and necrotizing agents in rats. *Food Chem Toxicol*. 1997, 35: 769–775.

60. Lorenz R, Weber PC, Szimnau P, Heldwein W, Strasser T, Loeschke K. Supplementation with n-3 fatty acids from fish oil in chronic inflammatory bowel disease—a randomized, placebo-controlled, double-blind cross-over trial. *J Intern Med Suppl*. 1989, 225: 225–232.

61. Lorenz R, Loeschke K. Placebo-controlled trials of omega 3 fatty acids in chronic inflammatory bowel disease. *World Rev Nutr Diet*. 1994, 76: 143–145.

62. Hollanders D, Tarnawski A. Is there a role for dietary essential fatty acids in gastroduodenal mucosal protection. *J Clin Gastroenterol.* 1991, 13: S72–S74.

63. Grant H, Palmer K, Riermesma R, Oliver M. Duodenal ulcer is associated with low dietary linoleic acid intake. *Gut.* 1989, 31: 997–998.

64. Al-Harbi M, Islam M, Al-Shabanah O, Al-Gharably N. Efect of acute administration of fish oil (omega-3 marine triglyceride) on gastric ulceration and secretion induced by various ulcerogenic and necrotizing agents in rats. *Fd Chem Toxic.* 1995, 33: 553–558.

65. Lin MY, Dipalma JA, Martini MC, Gross CJ, Harlander SK, Savaiano DA. Comparative effects of exogenous lactase (beta-galactosidase) preparations on in vivo lactose digestion. *Dig Dis Sci.* 1993, 38: 2022–2027.

66. Ramirez FC, Lee K, Graham DY. All lactase preparations are not the same: Results of a prospective, randomized, placebo-controlled trial. *Am J Gastroenterol.* 1994, 89: 566–570.

67. Lin MY, Yen CL, Chen SH. Management of lactose maldigestion by consuming milk containing lactobacilli. *Dig Dis Sci.* 1998, 43:133–137.

68. Jin LZ, Ho YW, Abdullah N, Jalaludin S. Digestive and bacterial enzyme activities in broilers fed diets supplemented with Lactobacillus cultures. *Poult Sci.* 2000, 79: 886–891.

69. Saltzman JR, Russell RM, Golner B, Barakat S, Dallal GE, Goldin BR. A randomized trial of *Lactobacillus acidophilus* BG2FO4 to treat lactose intolerance [see comments]. *Am J Clin Nutr.* 1999, 69: 140–146.

70. Mustapha A, Jiang T, Savaiano DA. Improvement of lactose digestion by humans following ingestion of unfermented acidophilus milk: Influence of bile sensitivity, lactose transport, and acid tolerance of *Lactobacillus acidophilus. J Dairy Sci.* 1997, 80: 1537–1545.

71. Savaiano DA, AbouElAnouar A, Smith DE, Levitt MD. Lactose malabsorption from yogurt, pasteurized yogurt, sweet acidophilus milk, and cultured milk in lactase-deficient individuals. *Am J Clin Nutr.* 1984, 40: 1219–1223.

72. Gebhardt R. Antioxidative and protective properties of extracts from leaves of the artichoke (Cynara scolymus L.) against hydroperoxide-induced oxidative stress in cultured rat hepatocytes. *Toxicol Appl Pharmacol.* 1997, 144: 279–286.

73. Englisch W, Beckers C, Unkauf M, Ruepp M, Zinserling V. Efficacy of Artichoke dry extract in patients with hyperlipoproteinemia. *Arzneimittelforschung.* 2000, 50: 260–265.

74. Brown JE, Rice-Evans CA. Luteolin-rich artichoke extract protects low density lipoprotein from oxidation in vitro. *Free Radic Res.* 1998, 29: 247–255.

75. Gebhardt R. Inhibition of cholesterol biosynthesis in primary cultured rat hepatocytes by artichoke (Cynara scolymus L.) extracts. *J Pharmacol Exp Ther.* 1998, 286: 1122–1128.

76. Kirchoff R, Beckers C, Kirchoff G, et al. Increase in choloresis by means of artichoke extract. *Phytomedicine.* 1994, 1: 107–115.

77. Kraft K. Artichoke leaf extract—recent findings reflecting effects on lipid metabolism, liver and gastrointestinal tracts. *Pytomedicine.* 1997, 4: 370–378.

78. Al-Habbal MJ, Al-Habbal Z, Huwez FU. A double-blind controlled clinical trial of mastic and placebo in the treatment of duodenal ulcer. *Clin Exp Pharmacol Physiol.* 1984, 11: 541–544.

79. Ekstrom AM, Serafini M, Nyren O, Hansson LE, Ye W, Wolk A. Dietary antioxidant intake and the risk of cardia cancer and noncardia cancer of the intestinal and diffuse types: A population-based case-control study in Sweden. *Int J Cancer.* 2000, 87: 133–140.

80. Huwez FU, Al-Habbal MJ. Mastic in treatment of benign gastric ulcers. *Gastroenterol Jpn.* 1986, 21: 273–274.

81. Iauk L, Ragusa S, Rapisarda A, Franco S, Nicolosi V. *In vitro* antimicrobial activity of *Pistacia lentiscus* L. extracts: Preliminary report. *J Chemotherapy.* 1996, 8: 207–209.

82. Tassou C, Nychas G. Antimicrobial activity of the essential oil of mastic gum (*Pistacia lentiscus* var *chia*) on gram positive and gram negative bacteria in broth and in model food system. 1995: 411–420.

83. Malekzadeh F. An antimicrobial compound in two *Pistacia* species. *Mycopathologia et Mycologia applicata.* 1974, 54: 73–77.

84. Huwez FU, Thirlwell D, Cockayne A, Ala'Aldeen DA. Mastic gum kills *Helicobacter pylori*. *N Engl J Med.* 1998, 339: 1946.

85. Al-Said MS, Ageel AM, Parmar NS, Tariq M. Evaluation of mastic, a crude drug obtained from *Pistacia lentiscus* for gastric and duodenal anti-ulcer activity. *J Ethnopharmacol.* 1986, 15: 271–278.

INDEX